Overcoming Abuse: Embracing Peace. What a treasure-trove of help and hope! This author tackles one of the toughest topics on Earth—the tragedy of abuse. Davison knows that most people throughout the world are ignorant about the why's of abuse and especially the what-to-do's.

The pervasiveness of domestic violence is appalling (1 in 3 women worldwide). The *prevalence of childhood sexual abuse is heartbreaking—we must intervene.*

Thankfully, these insightful pages are filled with a plethora of Scriptural principles and *practical strategies ready for us to apply—to set the captives free. Consequently, to help us and to help us help others, we all need these books.*

June Hunt
Broadcaster, Hope for the Heart
Author, *Counseling Through Your Bible Handbook*

Reina Davison provides essential hope to abuse victims and valuable guidance to those who counsel and care for them. Overcoming Abuse Embracing Peace Volume I, II, and III are unique contributions to the understanding and treatment of abuse trauma. These are must have tools for counselors, caregivers, and abuse sufferers alike.

Major General Bob Dees, U.S. Army, Retired
Author, *The Resilience Trilogy and Resilience God Style*

Reina Davison's books are shrouded in truth. I held my breath as I read *Overcoming Abuse: Embracing Peace* Volume I and II. It's a necessary, but painful topic and Davison handles it with grace, courage, and wisdom. Naming the abuse—calling unhealthy behaviors out for what they are—puts power, hope, and the possibility of healing into the hands of the victim and those who desire to help. Written in a forthright style, these books are must reads. They are steeped in honesty and compassion, giving readers ample opportunity to reflect on and apply what they are uncovering in the pages.

Vicki Tiede
Vicki Tiede Ministries
Author of *When Your Husband is Addicted to Pornography: Healing Your Wounded Heart*

If women and children are ever to count as equals with men -- and abuse is one of the pivotal matters --, the change must come about in our time. With this in mind, Reina Davison's *Overcoming Abuse: Embracing Peace* Volume I, II, and III strike us as a compassionate enterprise of the first importance. May it flourish for years to come.

Julia O'Faolain, Novelist
Lauro Martines, Historian

The subtitles for Reina Davison's books are not exaggerations. The word 'encyclopedic' is accurate. These *Overcoming Abuse* companion volumes I, II, and III provide helpers and victims alike with a wealth of important insights into the tragic problem of abusive relationships and how to deal with them.

Abuse is a difficult problem for churches and church leaders to address. In the first place, abuse is not as simple as it might seem to the casual observer. It is complex, secretive, and entrenched. Simple exhortations or solutions do little more than allow the abuse to continue. Second, while abuse has significant spiritual causes, the role of psychological and emotional factors requires deeper and more nuanced understanding. Abuse is not a problem for mere spiritual formation strategies. It requires a comprehensive and professional set of interventions before it will give way to peace and freedom for the victim. Third, the church has a long history of male-dominated leadership. One of the most tragic consequences of this gender imbalance is that well-intentioned 'helpers' in the church often give more credence to the reports of males than to the plaints of women. Too often the church blames the victim for the abuse without taking into consideration the entire scope of the issues involved.

These books contain first-person accounts of victims that grip your heart. The tragedy that these victims have endured is immense. Yet we can all learn by listening to their stories and taking their experiences seriously. The massive problem of abuse in relationships, even those within the church, require all of us to be informed and equipped to deal effectively with it. The Overcoming Abuse volumes go a long way to do just that.

James R. Beck, Ph.D.
Senior Professor of Counseling
Denver Seminary

Overcoming Abuse Embracing Peace

VOLUME II

YOUR ENCYCLOPEDIC GUIDE TO FREEDOM FROM ABUSE

Reina Davison

NEW HARBOR PRESS

Rapid City, SD

Copyright © 2020 by Reina Davison.

All rights reserved. No part of this publication may be reproduced, distributed or transmitted in any form or by any means, including photocopying, recording, or other electronic or mechanical methods, without the prior written permission of the publisher, except in the case of brief quotations embodied in critical reviews and certain other noncommercial uses permitted by copyright law. For permission requests, write to the publisher, addressed "Attention: Permissions Coordinator," at the address below.

Davison/New Harbor Press
1601 Mt. Rushmore Rd.
Rapid City, SD 57701
www.NewHarborPress.com

Ordering Information:
Quantity sales. Special discounts are available on quantity purchases by corporations, associations, and others. For details, contact the "Special Sales Department" at the address above.

Overcoming Abuse II/ Reina Davison —1st ed.
ISBN 978-1-63357-220-1

This book is a work of non-fiction. Unless otherwise noted, the author and the publisher make no explicit guarantees as to the accuracy of the information contained in this book and in some cases, names of people and places have been altered to protect their privacy. The information, ideas, and suggestions in this book are not intended as a substitute for professional advice. Before following any suggestions contained in this book, you should consult your personal physician or mental health professional. Neither the author nor the publisher shall be liable or responsible for any loss or damage allegedly arising as a consequence of your use or application of any information or suggestions in this book. Because of the dynamic nature of the Internet, any web addresses or links contained in this book may have changed since publication and may no longer be valid.

The author has researched data and sources which are believed to be reliable information that is in accordance with the professional code of ethics and current standards of practice at the time of publication. In the event of the possibility of human error or changes in the medical and mental health sciences, neither the author nor the editor and publisher, or any other parties who were involved in the process or publication of this book guarantees that the information contained in this work is complete and flawless in respect to accuracy and they are not responsible for accidental omissions, errors, or any outcomes which result from the use of the information in this book. Readers are encouraged to consult with Scripture, continue the research contained in this book, and to confirm with additional sources.

All Scripture quotations are taken from the New King James Version®. Copyright 1982 by Thomas Nelson, Inc. Used by permission. All rights reserved.

Cover art by Victoria Aleice
Author photo by Tessa Klingensmith

*Dedicated to my Heavenly Father,
Who created woman, and Whose
Word instructs that women are to be
loved as Christ loved the Church.*

Contents

FOREWORD 1
ACKNOWLEDGMENTS 5
NOTE ON SELECTED TERMINOLOGY 9
AN INVITATION FOR
THE BEST USE OF THESE BOOKS 15

PART I

SPIRIT MIND BODY 21
    Balancing Your Spirit 21
    Balancing Your Mind 52
    Balancing Your Body 76
    Spirit Mind & Body Covenant 108
CASSANDRE'S STORY 109

PART II

OVERCOMER PRINCIPLES 127
    Overcomer Defined 127
    How Does a Victim Become an *Overcomer?* 136
    Overcoming Abuse is a Choice 146

Post-Escape Safety Plan 147
Overcomer Characteristics 156
The *Overcomer* Lifestyle 158
An *Overcomer* has Purpose 162

GRACE'S STORY 167

PART III

EMBRACING PEACE 175

Surrendering Your Victimization 175
Receive His Peace 180
A Personal Relationship with God
Provides Peace 184
God Advocates for Your Peace 193
The Power of Humility & His Forgiveness 196
God's Love Restores You 200
God's Word Renders Peace 205
Accept His Peace 210

BASILIA'S STORY 217

Contents

PART IV
ENCOURAGEMENT
FOR THE VICTIM & *OVERCOMER* 233
   You Shall Overcome and be Led Out with Peace 233
CAROL'S STORY 245
ENDNOTES 257
RESOURCES 261
OTHER BOOKS BY REINA DAVISON 265

FOREWORD

WHEN REINA DAVISON INITIALLY asked me to provide a Foreword for the *Overcoming Abuse* book series, I was flattered, to be sure, but I did wonder quietly what our respective professions had in common, and how I could best introduce a book on a subject matter with which I was, mercifully, not terribly familiar. My career, after all, has been in the realm of clinical medicine, as a practitioner of Critical Care. For the better part of four decades, my days have been spent at the bedsides of the critically ill and dying in the intensive care unit of military and civilian hospitals. These patients are terribly ill, deeply broken physically and emotionally, and yes, spiritually. In many cases, their illness has befallen them because of inadvisable choices they have made in their lives; in others, illness has come unbidden, if you will, seemingly at random. Regardless, the devastation of their affliction is great, and their suffering, unknowable.

But clinically, I have not been acquainted with victims of abuse—or have I? Of course, I knew a few victims...a friend or a relative, one in particular, now long deceased (by suicide), about whose "situation" my mom had told me. And, "situations," as we called many things back then, were not openly discussed. Isn't that the case for many of us—we know *about* someone who is a victim of abuse, but not much more.

But Davison reassured me...she had heard me lecture on things medical through a spiritual lens; we have this much in common, that we trust in a Lord who is acquainted with grief and suffering, *our* grief and suffering, into which He entered, and enters, completely, and in which He is present to meet us and to be, finally, the only Source of healing and restoration.

Thus encouraged, I read the manuscripts—and it didn't take long before several dimensions of this work began to stand out. The first of these is Davison's breadth and depth of experience as a counselor and friend to the victims of abuse. She is a keen clinician, one who speaks authoritatively on her field of practice. She is knowledgeable in the subject of abuse, perceptive of the nuances of the illness, and familiar with pertinent literature on the subject. Like an astute physician, she is not fooled by the nuances of victims' symptoms, nor by the subconsciously illusive turns of the history that the abused will give, nor by the psychopathology of the abuser. Nor by the shroud of, well, frank *ignorance and denial* of abuse, which is individually and societally symptomatic of the disease itself and of its deep evil.

So it began to dawn on me that her line of work is not terribly divergent, after all, from my own. Victims of abuse are critically ill, and desperately so, and in need of their own form of *intensive care*. Davison provides precisely that: care for the victim and a resource for those who would care for them. And, like any great advocate, she is an educator—not only of the victim and their counselors, but of her readers. These books are nothing short of revelatory for those of us who, hitherto, "may only have known about" a victim, whether because we did not know the signs or manifestations, or because these were "situations" about which one doesn't speak. Perhaps *I have* met a number of people—

friend, relative, or patient—who have been victims, secretly suffering, and I never knew, because I hadn't been aware. These books raise consciousness.

The second dimension that caught my eye was Davison's faithfulness to the biblical teaching of the redemptive work of Christ and of the active and very real presence of the Holy Spirit to heal and restore. Davison's text is punctuated with the personal accounts of victims. Their path to healing is never "fake," as in the well caricatured tossing away of a no-longer-needed set of crutches, but of the complex, often tedious, but fundamentally important healing process that occurs over time and as a result of sound therapy, patience, and much prayer. The Holy Spirit is no less present and active in these long and difficult processes than in the dramatic healing of the paralytic at the Beautiful Gate (Acts 3:1-10). Davison's is not an appeal to a vague secular "spirituality," but to the mighty Triune God. The hope she offers is rock-solid.

The third key dimension of these books for me is their inherent and urgent relevance for the Church. It has always been incumbent upon the Church universal and the Church local to be sensitive and responsive to the deep brokenness of her members. Inasmuch as the Apostle Paul understands the institution of marriage itself to be the visible symbol of Christ and His church (Ephesians 5:32), we see perhaps no greater consequence of the fall of humankind than abuse, marital discord, dysfunction, and rupture. But do some churches strain to keep a marriage intact at the expense of the well-being or even the life of a victim of abuse? Davison is not shy to address this head-on. If the recognition, diagnosis, intervention, and counsel of abuse victims are not on the heart and in the pastoral care ministry of a church, then that church has work to do. Davison's books should find their way onto every pastor's desk, and into seminary curricula.

Ministry to victim and to abuser, like medical treatment of critically ill patients, is not for the faint of heart. Ministry and treatment are all about the rolling up of the sleeves of our hearts and minds, the speaking openly about the unspeakable, and entering into the thick darkness of compassion as we come alongside victims and abusers in the hard work of redemption, remembering, all the while, that thick darkness is the very place where God Himself is known to dwell. The prayers of the afflicted do certainly rise to the throne of God. Reina Davison has given practical wisdom of life and hope to those who are in deep and abiding need.

Allen H. Roberts II, M.D., M.Div., M.A. (Bioethics)
Professor of Clinical Medicine
Georgetown University Medical Center

ACKNOWLEDGMENTS

A HEARTFELT THANK YOU to the abusers and victims of whom these books are written; it is regrettable that there had to be abusers and victims for these books to be written, but the hope is that out of these tragic abusive relationships, victims will be reached and many lives will be saved. A wholehearted thank you to each Overcomer for responding in a humanitarian way by pouring out your heart and allowing your story to be shared in these books.

Thank you, colleagues—too many to acknowledge, but you know who you are because you sacrificially gave of your time to disclose your professional experiences in the community, with the government, the judicial system, with abusers and the victims of abuse.

Thank you, Hershall Seals, for taking time out of your schedule on some beautiful summer days and actually painting alongside Victoria Aleice on your own canvas as she created the covers for Volume I, II, and III, of the *Overcoming Abuse: Embracing Peace* book series. Thank you, Victoria Aleice, for painting the book covers with the exact vision I proposed to you; an oil painting with purple clouds (as purple is the official color for domestic violence awareness) depicting the darkness of the trauma of abuse on the bottom which then flows into an ombre lavender, fading into white clouds and sun (SON) rays streaming down at the top to represent the healing from darkness (abuse victim trauma) that turns into light (an Overcomer light of Christ).

Thank you, Dr. Roberts, for taking time out of your busy life to meticulously research and read the manuscripts for the *Overcoming Abuse: Embracing Peace* book series, and then writing a foreword. Thank you for caring about this ministry medically, educationally, and spiritually.

Thank you, Mary Ellis Rice, for poring over the *Overcoming Abuse: Embracing Peace* manuscripts and for proofreading, along with providing your welcomed suggested edits. From day one, in spite of your full agenda, you cared about the mission of this project and up until the day that you returned the manuscripts to me—you fulfilled what you said, "I want to do my best work."

To the New Harbor Press publishing assistants. My heart wells up with gratitude toward the thought of each of you being called to do this work for the abused, many years ago; before I even knew of you. As we all know, nothing is a surprise to our Master. The fact that each of you as a team member has been divinely appointed to be a part of this project was orchestrated long ago. I respect your gifts and servanthood toward this ministerial work. I am certain that there are others that unbeknownst to me are or will be a part of the production and delivery of these books and for them I am also grateful. However, I want to take a moment right now to recognize those that I am aware of who have contributed to this work. Thank you Rick Bates-Managing Editor, Pauline Harris-Editor, Steve Nordstrom-Project Manager, Bob Swanson-Typesetting, and Graphic Designer-Natalie Reed. May your service to the abused and helpers of the abused be rewarded a hundredfold!

ACKNOWLEDGMENTS

Thank you to all of my educational, clinical, and spiritual mentors past and present who have selflessly given of your time, wisdom, planted seeds in me, trained and coached me. Your mentoring is an eternal gift which I will treasure and continue to pass on.

My deep appreciation goes to my family of origin, and a tribute to my late parents for their influence in my life. I'm grateful to my immediate family and dear friends who have supported the writing of these books by lovingly standing back, allowing me the flexibility and space, and for praying, so that God's perfect timing would develop the books.

NOTE ON SELECTED TERMINOLOGY

For the purpose of readability and in an effort to select short universal terms, I have elected to use the words *abuse*, *abuser*, *spouse*, and *victim*. Abuse is used as a term that can involve all forms and levels of victim and family violence: emotional, physical, sexual, economic, and spiritual. This book is not intended to be offensively sexist when the male gender is referred to as the abuser and the female gender is referred to as the victim. My true desire and motive for this book is that it becomes a manual for the victim and any person that is interested in helping with the devastation of family violence.

To maintain a clear and simple discussion throughout the book, I at times refer to the husband or wife as the *spouse*. When referring to the *perpetrator*, I have selected the shorter term, *abuser*, not because I believe that every man who has problems with controlling behaviors is an abuser, but because it is a word that applies to any man who has consistent, ongoing problems with disrespecting, devaluing, and controlling behaviors toward his spouse.

When I refer to a spouse it's not to imply that premarital abuse doesn't exist; in most cases the abuse begins *before* the marriage and goes undetected or ignored until the consummation of the marriage. I have elected to use the term *he* to refer to the abusive spouse. This is not about denigrating men—it's the *mindset* of abusive men that the research addresses, not their manhood. The term *he* is used because the term describes the majority of the research done on relationships in which power and control are misused by men. The research in the June 28, 2013 U.S. Department of Justice, Bureau of Justice Statistics Report documented ninety-five percent of victims of domestic violence are women.

When writing about the woman that is being abused, I use the term *victim,* not because I view that woman as a helpless dupe but because it is a term that applies to any woman suffering from some act(s) of violence that has led her to have severe recurring feelings of intimidation, humiliation, confusion, anxiousness, fear, and/or depression. In selecting women as my victimization sample, it is not to infer that men are not abused.

If you are a man that is in an abusive relationship with your wife, there is information in this book for you as well. Wives that abuse their husbands share the same socialization, background, history, and dynamics as abusive men do. Female abusers use the same tactics, rationalizations, and excuses for their behavior as male abusers. Husbands that are consistently abused by their wives have the same characteristics as wives that are victims of abuse. So read on; you will just have to change the gender language to fit your experience as an abused husband.

In order to incorporate every potential counselor (that may have an opportunity to work with family violence), I have selected the term *professional* or simultaneously the word *helper* as

NOTE ON SELECTED TERMINOLOGY

opposed to using the title of each mental health practitioner and clergy member. The word "professional" is not used to infer that laypeople are not capable of ministering or working professionally with victims of abuse. The "professional" or "helper" is referred to in the masculine pronoun for the sake of uniformity and word simplicity (applies to both female and male professionals).

The narrative stories that are recounted in this book are all authentic. They are the victims' personal experiences and perceptions of abuse, as told to this writer. They are offered for the victim to recognize and easily identify the various types of abuse via another victim's story; and for the victim to be inspired and encouraged that she too can be healed from the trauma of abuse. Each story has their given name left out, and the victim (now an *Overcomer*) has selected a name with which to be identified. For her protection and privacy, other identifying factors are not disclosed.

The abuser's name and all identifying data have been changed. Any similarities to a reader or circumstances of an individual are simply a resemblance as each of these biographies have been tape recorded, reviewed by the subject, and documented for publication with the subject's signed consent. Permission has been obtained from all research study subjects and case scenario examples cited in this book; if any similarities are recognized, it is purely coincidental. The color purple is the official, symbolic color for family violence; it is used in the book cover, in memory of those victims known and unknown that have been killed by their abusers.

The name "God," His proper names, and pronouns referring to God are capitalized out of reverence to Him. Since capitalization is like italicization—it's a method that suggests "importance" and emphasis—I have elected not to extol satan's name, thus his name is not capitalized. Because God the Father, God the Son, and God the Holy Spirit are One in the same trinity,

I am referring to the three of them simultaneously when I'm speaking of our Heavenly Father, since they are each equal as one God (Genesis 1:1-2, 1 John 5:7, John 10:30, Matthew 3:16-17, Matthew 28: 18-19, 2 Corinthians 13:14).

The word *Overcomer* is capitalized as a proper noun and given importance because the word represents Jesus; it is also set apart from the other text for emphasis. All Scriptural quotations are from The Holy Bible, New King James Version. The same Scriptural references may be quoted in parts of this book in order to expand on the verse, use it in a different context, or facilitate comprehension through a different example.

When referring to the victim's *soul,* I am referring to her emotional and moral sense of identity. When speaking of the victim's immaterial being, which is the nerve center for her feelings and sentiments, I speak of her *heart.* I am not using the term soul in a theological form as her immortal part of her being. Conversely, when I refer to her spirit, I am then speaking about her mood or immortal and eternal soul. The Spirit (Holy Spirit) is always capitalized.

The term *mindful* is used to describe the process of becoming aware of one's thinking as related to the mental technique of *mindfulness,* not as in a religious ritual, but as conscious mindful observations of one's thoughts, experiences, and behaviors.

It is a tough calling to comprehensively document years of observing and working with the lives of victims and abusers, and it is even tougher to write in a language that depicts their life through their eyes.

Those of us therapists and others who write about the taboo subject of abuse and report the darkness and the evil that victims encounter dare to open Pandora's Box and risk public scrutiny and credibility in the same way as the victim. To speak and transparently write about the devouring consequences of

NOTE ON SELECTED TERMINOLOGY

abuse trauma in a society that silences victims of abuse invites controversy.

It has been my sincere desire throughout the writing of this book to put into words only the precise expressions and descriptions from the dialogues of the victim, abuser, and society—to depict what I've listened to, witnessed, and worked with.

> "May He grant you according to your heart's *desire*,
> And fulfill all your purpose.
> May the Lord fulfill all your petitions."
> Psalm 20:4

AN INVITATION FOR THE BEST USE OF THESE BOOKS

The Overcoming Abuse Volume I, II, and III encyclopedic guidebooks were created through the work done with individuals experiencing the dynamics of family abuse. My clinical sources for these books are the victim and the abuser. Both my research and experience with these soldiers, clients, inmates, and patients have consistently indicated the same end results: No matter what class, cultural, ethnic, or racial background they come from, the dynamics of the victim of abuse remain the same; the dynamics for the abuser are consistently the same. There are universal characteristics among the hundreds of victims and abusers that my colleagues and I have researched and worked with in the past four decades. Samples of case scenarios from victims who have willingly voiced their stories of abuse are included at the end of each part of the books to encourage you so that you too can overcome your abuse! So you too, can help the abused.

It is my intent to share in these books a body of knowledge on the trauma of abuse. My goal is to encourage women in abusive relationships to receive this message: that there is hope, and that the cycle of abuse can be stopped *before* it begins with the next generation. The purpose of these encyclopedic guidebooks is to empower women who are involved in an abusive relationship into permanent recovery—to be set free from the cycle of abuse and their abuser. These books teach women how to identify an abuser in order to prevent them from getting involved in an abusive relationship(s) again. Secondly, imbedded in that effort is my goal to empower families and our society as a whole with an awareness and understanding of family violence through education on the trauma of abuse.

Will the abuser be happy that the victim is reading these books? Absolutely not, so these books are best kept a secret between the victim and her support system. There are good and bad secrets to keep; this is a good secret to keep. Whether you have the books in electronic copy or in book form, you must take safety precautions in preserving the books. It may be easier/safer for you to download your book to your tablet or into your TracFone smart phone (see Resources for TracFone information). If you feel that you can't maintain a private password for your e-books or that you have no private place to keep a copy of these books in your home, rather than living in fear that your abuser will discover them, take them to work. If that's not an option and you feel most comfortable asking someone to store them for you, then ask a friend. Or, put book covers on them and ask your church secretary/librarian if you can confidentially keep them in an undisturbed area at the church (be creative!).

If you are uncertain as to whether your spouse's behavior should be classified as abusive, glance through Volume I Part I of

AN INVITATION FOR THE BEST USE OF THESE BOOKS

this book, which can help to clarify the definition of abuse. Even if your spouse's behavior doesn't fit the definition of abuse, if your spouse is consistently controlling and disrespectful, there is still a problem. Having a disrespectful and controlling relationship with your spouse is a problem. Controlling spouses fall on a range of behavioral tactics (as discussed in Volume I Part II Abuser Characteristics) from exhibiting only *some* tactics to exhibiting *most* of them. All the recurring thoughts and feelings that a victim experiences may still have an unhealthy effect. Abuse ranges from *mild* to *severe*; nevertheless, all abuse has the same impact on the victim (See Volume I Part III, Victim Characteristics). Additionally, examples of abusive relationships are cited throughout the books with stories of women who were once victims of abuse but now lead recovered lives—free from abuse. These stories are case scenarios that will not only help you to answer the question of whether your spouse's behavior is abusive, but they will also encourage you to realize that abuse is a preventable and treatable health problem which you can overcome!

Not all of the information written in these books will pertain to your abusive relationship. If there are parts of the books in which I describe the abuser or the victim, and those parts do not fit or apply to you or your relationship, it's alright to skip to the part that does apply. Not everyone has the same lifestyle; read what is most helpful to *your* specific circumstances or abusive relationship. I do not wish at any point in these books to cause you discomfort by telling you how your situation is. You are already bombarded with mind-control games; you don't need another person to tell you how you should think or act. I don't want to become a part of that very unhealthy pattern to which you have been subjected.

At the same time, I do not recommend that you skim read the books, as this can lead to a misinterpretation of the contents and message. Use each book as a guideline. Listen to what our Heavenly Father has inspired me to write and you to read. If it doesn't speak to you or your situation and does not re-create the abusive dynamics as they are played out in the particulars of your household, it doesn't apply. These books are structured in an encyclopedic topical form to allow you to identify the information you are searching for and to refer back to the sections that you can read later. They were created to conveniently accommodate an opportunity for you to access information quickly if you are in a crisis state.

Even if you skip the parts that do not apply, one truth does remain the same for all households that experience abuse: an abuser will alter your lifestyle and your mind so that *everything* becomes focused on him. The strategic way out of this abusive torment is to take charge of your person! Focus on you, and if children are involved, your children's well-being as well. It is imperative that you reclaim your person, stop dwelling on your abuser, and instead use that energy to *overcome* your abuse. Overcoming abuse is a daunting journey. I say it is a journey, not to further stress you, or to suggest that it is a never-ending rite of passage, but to communicate to you that it is a *process*. Processes that can, miraculously through supernatural power, evolve—and can be resolved! You must no longer carry this burden of an abusive relationship alone. The Lord invites you to lighten your burden (actually commands you to unburden yourself) when He says, "Take My yoke upon you and learn from Me, for I am gentle and lowly in heart, and you will find rest for your souls. For My yoke *is* easy and My burden is light" (Matthew 11:29-30). Our burdens are made lighter through His companionship!

After confiding in the Lord—the Good Shepherd ("I am the good shepherd." John 10:11a, "The LORD *is* my Shepherd; I shall not want" Psalm 23:1), you must follow up by confiding in *someone else* about your abusive relationship. It is like getting

AN INVITATION FOR THE BEST USE OF THESE BOOKS

an under-shepherd (a supportive assistant). If the sheriff has an undersheriff (deputy), so can you! Confiding in the Good Shepherd and someone else provides you with an under-shepherd; it is your first step to getting free and overcoming abuse.

You may feel guilty for speaking negatively to anyone about your spouse or ashamed of your spouse's abusive behavior. You may fear the person whom you tell will scrutinize you as to *why* you continue to tolerate this abuse. Perhaps the concern may be that you will not be believed because, after all, your spouse is such a hard-working family man in the eyes of the Church, employer, or his community. Regardless, in order to *heal* and to obtain *peace*, surrendering your abusive burden to the Lord and seeking support while reading these books is absolutely *necessary*. Some women (particularly those that have been coerced into near isolation) will feel extremely uncomfortable reading these books, which may generate unbearable feelings that have unconsciously or consciously been blocked. These books may initiate leaving the comfort zone of *denial* when overwhelming realizations about your abuse are brought to the surface. In spite of the fact that your trust level is tender and has been violated by those that have abused you, I still highly recommend that you consider contacting someone you trust, as an *under-shepherd*. If it's safe, reach out to this trustworthy person.

Pray about who that person may be, and then make the contact. This person may be a friend, family member, pastor, pastor's wife, church member, counselor, or an organization (organizations are listed under "Resources" at the end of this book). I realize *trusting* someone as a support system is extremely difficult for some women because there is a *fear* of the reaction and judgment from that person (when you tell them your secrets about being mistreated by your spouse). However, having a support system is a *vital* part of problem-solving and accountability.

Having this support will expedite your healing process in overcoming your abuse.

Consequently, these books are written in three volumes. Volumes I and II are written for you—the abused. Volume III is for lay people and those in the helping professions who are the support system for victims of abuse. There is no rule that you as a recovering victim of abuse cannot proceed to read Volume III; vice versa, if a helper wants to grow in the knowledge of the dynamics of abuse, the abuser profile, and the characteristics of victims of abuse, he/she can read Volume I and II.

So, let's move forward on this journey to overcome your abuse!

> **"God *is* with you in all that you do."**
> **Genesis 21:22**

PART I

SPIRIT MIND BODY

Balancing Your Spirit
IN OVERCOMING ABUSE VOLUME I your Spirit, Mind, and Body was saturated and strengthened with hope to overcome your abuse. We learned the descriptive definitions of various types of abuse and abuse trauma. We unveiled the abuser profile, his inveterate behavioral problem of abuse (sin) and why he chooses not to change. Together, we uncovered the characteristics of the victim, why she stays; and we explored some of the virtues of an Overcomer. In unison we developed a personal Safety Escape Plan (SEP) and now in Volume II as a part of recovery we will create a Post-Escape Plan (PESP). Volume I concluded with the admonishment that to overcome your abuse or help someone overcome abuse trauma; inaction is not an option. You were left with a reassurance that God and you are capable of overcoming and that it is paramount to overcoming your past and present abuse; that you move forward if you are to experience freedom from abuse and live in peace.

Abuse means living under chronic stress. Stress is generally described as the rate of cognitive, emotional, physical and spiritual adjustments/changes your body has to endure and make as you respond or react to demands, pressures, and daily vacillating circumstances in your life. When a person's stressors are greater than their coping skills, support, and/or resources; the results are high levels of anxiety and hopelessness. Anxiety affects the Spirit, Mind, and Body. Volume II proceeds with our goal and plan to overcome your abuse by leading you to embrace peace through learning to guide your life onward to an abuse-free balanced state; via your Spirit, Mind, and Body. The dimensions of an Overcomer's well-being are the Spirit, Mind, and Body (in that order).

As we continue this journey to your freedom from abuse you will become increasingly aware that for the victim of abuse staying spiritually, emotionally, and physically safe is a weary full-time job. However, as a recovered Overcomer you will find that being free from abuse is a blessed divine deployment and employment: a pleasantry of insightful expectation of actually receiving and experiencing healing peace. An experience the Overcomer does not grow weary of! Let's begin our study of the Spirit, Mind, and Body.

Some practitioners in the healthcare field encourage the alignment of the *body*, *mind*, and *spirit* in that order, which is a holistic approach to our well-being. I believe in and am in favor of a holistic approach in the treatment of the patient; however, I elect to align a person's well-being in the order of the Spirit, Mind, and Body for reasons that I articulate in this part of the book.

Whenever I refer to the Spirit, I am not referring to secular spirituality. Secular spirituality adheres to the person's spirit being one without a relationship with God, the inner peace that comes from the individual. Secular spirituality focuses on humanistic qualities without divine intervention. Secular spirituality relies totally on the person nurturing their own thoughts, emotions, and actions without the supernatural power of God. The Spirit that I refer to and work with as a Christian therapist is the Holy Spirit, Who is capable of dwelling within each human being.

> "Do you not know that you are the temple of God and *that* the Spirit of God dwells in you? If anyone defiles the temple of God, God will destroy him. For the temple of God is holy, which *temple* you are" (1Corinthians 3:16-17).

The Spirit, Mind, and Body are entwined; what influences one influences the others. There is much research that has been done through alternative medicine which indicates that there is a connection between disease and an imbalance among a patient's physical, emotional, spiritual, and environmental elements.

I am all for a holistic treatment plan for a victim or any other patient. But I am not in concurrence with the idea that people ought to look within themselves for human power as their own God. I elect to treat the Spirit, Mind, and Body; traditional therapists elect to treat symptoms with medication and psychoanalysis or other psychological theories. My preference is to look at what is *causing* the symptoms and go beyond exploring the mind on the surface. I reserve recommending therapeutic drugs as a last option *unless* acute mental illness is the primary diagnosis and other treatment modalities have already been used. Recommending therapeutic drugs does not seek to resolve the underlying causes of the symptoms and only conceals the symptoms. While reducing symptoms with therapeutic drugs may be a temporary solution for *some* patients, it leaves serious underlying problems unresolved.

Holistic approaches encourage the alignment of the body, mind, and spirit, separately. When the Spirit is not connected to the mind and body, the person feels defenseless with the disorder in their life. The Spirit is the driving force behind the mind *and* body, the driving force behind the person's life. When the mind and body are placed before the Spirit, they war against the person's Spirit. This is because of what Proverbs 23:7 says is the case: as a man thinks in his heart, so is he. Using the Spirit to renew the mind and discipline the body is essential—because the condition of the mind is the condition of one's heart. When one's heart is in order, so are one's thinking and actions. I elect to place the Spirit first when using a holistic approach in treatment because when the patient aligns their Spirit with their mind and body (in that order), that person's entire perspective on the self, others, and life changes! That person is now on their way to find their meaning and purpose for their life.

Caution—many individuals that have never had a personal encounter with the Spirit will be uncomfortable, and they may even act with an underlying allegation that the person experiencing the Spirit is crazy! These individuals may even act offensively toward the person that has activated the Spirit within them and, out of ignorance, decide to speak no further with the person on the matters of the Spirit. Regardless, these individuals in your life need to be treated with respect in spite of their rejection of the Spirit's existence. Some of these individuals may even defensively use sarcasm or mock you for acknowledging the presence of the Spirit within you; they may even call you, who is speaking based on your belief in Christ and the Holy Spirit, a "religious fanatic."

We all have a choice to either use the Spirit that lives within us or not. Those who have made a clear choice *not* to believe in the Spirit are to be treated in the same way as if they recognized the Spirit because it is just a matter of their being unable to understand the things of the Spirit at this time. The following Scriptures speak on how the Holy Spirit operates within each of us: "However, when He, the Spirit of truth, has come, He will guide you into all truth; for He will not speak on His own *authority*, but whatever He hears He will speak; and He will tell you things to come" (John 16:13). "But the natural man does not receive the things of the Spirit of God, for they are foolishness to him; nor can he know *them*, because they are spiritually discerned" (1 Corinthians 2:14). "For the message of the cross is foolishness to those who are perishing, but to us who are being saved it is the power of God" (1 Corinthians 1:18). Our intellect is insufficient to understand spiritual matters because spiritual things can only be discerned by the Holy Spirit. When you are led by the Holy Spirit, you are inspired into thinking, feeling, or action; inspiration comes from the Spirit. The word *inspiration* itself means to be *in spirit*.

At this point, it merits discussing *how* a person can actively receive the Spirit of God within. It's one of the simplest acts that a human being can do—ask God (the Holy Spirit) to come into their heart. All you have to do is *believe*, and the power of the Holy Spirit will come to you! This then allows you to start a new life with Christ in your heart. It's also called being born-again because the person now has embarked on a new life in Christ. "Therefore, if anyone *is* in Christ, *he is* a new creation; old things have passed away; behold, all things have become new" (2 Corinthians 5:17). Why in the world would a victim, or *any* human being for that matter, need to be born again? Why does *everyone* need to be born again? This question is actually answered in the Bible: "Jesus answered and said to him, "'Most assuredly, I say to you, unless one is born again, he cannot see the kingdom of God'" (John 3:3). What does it *mean* to be "born again?" To be born again is to be *Spiritually* born again, not as a religious ritualistic act but to be born again as Christ calls us to be, in the Bible. It means to have the Holy Spirit born in you.

Being born of the Spirit or being born again simply means that you have an opportunity to be *born twice*. Your first birth is your physical birth through your parents; you are born into their family. The second birth is your Spiritual birth (born again). Your Spiritual birth means being born again when Jesus Christ is born in you and literally comes into your body to reside in the form of the Holy Spirit (the Spirit of God). Being born again is the same as when in the Bible, the apostles were filled with the Holy Spirit. Jesus said, "Receive the Holy Spirit" (John 20:22). He will send His Spirit into your heart so that you may grow only the fruit (including peace) that befits your *Overcomer* conversion. Once the Holy Spirit ascends upon you, God *recognizes you* from heaven as one of His children for whom He has granted a life of eternal *peace*! Being born again means you are Spiritually reborn into a new family—God's family. Being born again means you have now inherited becoming a part of one of the most privileged families on Earth—Christ's family!

> "And I will pray the Father, and He will give you another Helper, that He may abide with you forever— the Spirit of truth, whom the world cannot receive, because it neither sees Him nor knows Him; but you know Him, for He dwells with you and will be in you. I will not leave you orphans; I will come to you" (John 14:16-18).

Our bodies are spiritually dead until we receive the Holy Spirit (James 2:26). "It is the Spirit who gives life; the flesh profits nothing. The words that I speak to you are spirit, and *they* are life" (John 6:63). Our spirit is dead upon birth because our spirit is dead in sin; we are born without Jesus (God) in us, as we are born from the inheritance of Adam and Eve who sinned against God. Once born, we're all given a free will to choose to remain dead in sin or to receive His Spirit, live, and spend eternity with Him. Free will places the responsibility on us for whom we allow to lead us; we can be led by our own human spirit or by the power of our divine Spirit. We can yield and become a slave to our human spirit or obey God and yield to His Spirit within us. Yielding to your frail, fleshly spirit by thinking, "Oh, I've got this, I'm going to fix it and things will get better," only leads to the abuse dominating you because you chose willingly to yield to it (through submission to your carnal spirit).

> "For those who live according to the flesh set their minds on the things of the flesh, but those *who live* according to the Spirit, the things of the Spirit. For to be carnally minded *is* death, but to be spiritually minded *is* life and peace. So then, those who are in the flesh cannot please God. But you are not in the flesh but in the Spirit, if indeed the Spirit of God dwells in you. Now if anyone does not have the Spirit of Christ, he is not His" (Romans 8:5-6, 8-9).

Yielding to your human spirit can become an enchaining experience. The human spirit has no power to break the bondage of abuse trauma; yielding to your human soul makes you a bond slave to yourself. Yielding to the Spirit of God means having the power to break every form of dysfunctional slavery—including abuse. "Do you not know that to whom you present yourselves slaves to obey, you are that one's slaves whom you obey, whether of sin *leading* to death, or of obedience *leading* to righteousness?" (Romans 6:16). When you invite the Spirit of God to indwell within you, satan's stronghold on your life is invaded and defeated; you can then proceed to join God as He actualizes His plans of peace for your life. Nothing, not satan or any other dark inferno, can put out the light of the Spirit of God within you—once your human spirit has accepted the Spirit of God, it is an eternal, inextinguishable light.

We humans were created in the same image as Jesus Christ in the form of a body and spirit. "But he who is joined to the Lord is one spirit *with Him*. Or do you not know that your body is the temple of the Holy Spirit *who is* in you, whom you have from God, and you are not your own?" (1 Corinthians 6:17, 19). Our Spirit returns to God when we die. "Then the dust will return to the earth as it was, and the spirit will return to God who gave it" (Ecclesiastes 12:7).

A victim, through *free will*, gets to choose if she wants to remain spiritually dead or if she wants to receive the Holy Spirit (to be spiritually born again) and allow Jesus to infill her with His Spirit. When a victim receives the Holy Spirit, she is *saved* from spending eternity where spiritually dead people go after their body dies—hell. Not having fellowship with Jesus is like having "bad blood" (discord in a family relationship). Accepting Jesus develops or restores your relationship with God; bad blood becomes a part of your past. Inviting Jesus into your heart is like getting a blood transfusion; you receive Him because He gives His shed blood for you. You're in His bloodline now—you're part of God's family when you accept Him. Jesus offers the invitation to receive His Spirit and to spend one's life eternally in heaven with Him, but He *never forces anyone* to accept Him as their Savior. Offering to receive His spirit is a part of His plan for one's *salvation*; He only asks that we confess our sins so that we may be forgiven and be ready to receive the purity of His Spirit. My economics professor said that in life, "there's no free lunch," meaning that nothing in life is free of cost. I'd like to disagree with him right now; there is one thing that *is* for free in this world and that is salvation. It *is a free* gift! "For the wages of sin *is* death, but the gift of God *is* eternal life in Christ Jesus our Lord" (Romans 6:23).

The victim or any one of us does not have to pay a price to receive the Spirit of God and salvation from hell; Jesus already paid the cost when humanity sinned against Him beforehand and crucified Him on the cross. We can continue in our lives with this inheritance of a sinful nature, or we can repent and ask God to forgive us for *all* of our past sins and accept His Spirit and be *saved* from being cast into hell when we die. Being born again (saved) is a very simple process. We're *saved* not just based on the repenting of our sins, but we are also saved simply by repenting of our unbelief of the gospel (the Bible). The Bible says that if we believe that Jesus died, was buried, and was raised from death, we are saved. "So they said, 'Believe on the Lord Jesus Christ, and you will be saved, you and your household'" (Acts 16:31). What happens if you don't believe? The answer to this question is the same throughout the Bible, such as in John 3:36: "He who believes in the Son has everlasting life; and he who does not believe the Son shall not see life, but the wrath of God abides on him." I leave you with food for thought on this question of belief. If you believe in the law of gravity or the feeling of love (which are invisible and you can't see), then it's the same approach to believing in the unseen: God the Father, Son, and Holy Spirit. We can experience the force of gravity and a love attraction, but we can't *see* the force itself.

Why should a victim consider that one of her tasks in her recovery from abuse is to accept the Holy Spirit? Because when a person *by faith* accepts Christ and His plan of salvation, that person is now born of God, and this then accelerates the process and guarantees her becoming an *Overcomer*. God promises that those who have faith and believe that Christ is His Son who died for our sins can have *Overcomer* victory. "For whatever is born of God overcomes the world. And this is the victory that has overcome the world—our faith. Who is he who overcomes the world, but he who believes that Jesus is the Son of God?" (1 John 5:4-5). (More on this in Part II *Overcomer* Principles).

A person who accepts Christ is *actually* reclaiming a relationship with the God Who created that person; their Heavenly Father can *now* claim their status as a child of God. If a person is considering God as a part of their living, or a part of their treatment process, the Holy Spirit cannot be ignored, overlooked, or debated because He *is* God. When a person is born again, they become a whole new person in Christ at that very moment that they place their faith in Him. That person loses their desire to live in their old sinful ways; as they live their new life in Christ. "Therefore, if anyone *is* in Christ, *he is* a new creation; old things have passed away; behold, all things have become new" (2 Corinthians 5:17). So then, what does salvation have to offer that you don't already have? Salvation offers freedom from the darkness and destruction that sin brings into one's life and ends the fear of death, resulting in exultant joy even amid the problems we encounter in this life.

Furthermore, the Bible teaches us that if we accept and receive the Holy Spirit, we are infilled with His *peace*. Once His Holy Spirit is accepted, God's Word proves its effectiveness in the person's life. It's through His Holy Spirit that you will be able to live your life in spiritual peace. When the Holy Spirit enters your heart, He brings wholeness within which provides His peace. This is because His forgiveness brings His *peace* into your relationship with God, yourself, and others. This is not a quasi or pseudo peace which the world talks about. The penetration of true, divine peace in our soul replaces our human non-peaceable self. Real peace can only be derived from the Spirit within because it is only when the Holy Spirit enters the heart of a human that peace can be born. And then, it is only when His trinity becomes Master of that human heart that true peace can be experienced. When you receive the Holy Spirit, your brokenness is healed and your eyes are opened and introduced to your true God, the true you, and the world as He created it, giving you a renewed perspective in your life, others' lives, and the many purposes and aspects of life that you may not have previously considered.

The Holy Spirit has to be turned on in order to receive His power. If He is turned off, then He cannot be assessed—He becomes like an uncharged cellphone: useless. You may want to ignore God and His Holy Spirit right now and upgrade your excuses for unbelief and rejection of Him, but remember you will still have to reckon with God at the end of your life. Will He be smiling and saying, "Well done, good and faithful daughter?" Or, will He not be greeting you in heaven? Should you decide to accept Him today, you then have His promise of His presence in both your Earthly and eternal life with Him!

Who is and what is the purpose of the Holy Spirit anyway? The attributes of the Holy Spirit and His purposes are beyond the framework of this book, but in the Bible, you will find some answers including that He is Truth, serves to discern and influence decision-making, and convicts right from wrong; He's a guide, advocate, a reference point, companion, a teacher, a counselor, helper, comforter, and reminder, and He brings love and peace to us and glory to the Father and Son. If you allow the Holy Spirit into your heart and quietly listen for His still, small voice, He will teach you while you walk in His Spirit; He will empower and strengthen you. He will lead you to many new truths about God, you, and your circumstances. "Be still and know that I *am* God" (Psalm 46:10a). He promises to "show you great and mighty things, which you do not know" (Jeremiah 33:3b).

Accepting the Holy Spirit means making a full-time commitment to God; it is a long-term conscious decision. For the victim to live for herself only (whether in happiness or sadness) requires zilch effort on her behalf and only delivers temporary satisfaction with no eternal value. A commitment to God the Father, Son, and Holy Spirit means she will live on a higher daily, eternal, spiritual plane. For a victim, receiving the power of the Holy Spirit is not a spiritual luxury; it becomes an urgent need if she desires to overcome her abuse. A personal relationship with Christ via the Holy Spirit is different than following a book with a theological formula or being a part of a religious organization. In the proper context, theological books and religious affiliations are tools for growth; but it's not the same as the power of the work of the Holy Spirit Who can convert a victim into an *Overcomer*. There's no comparison with the victim's own strength to the unparalleled Holy Spirit guidance and energy the victim receives. Relying solely on her strength only leads to frustration, discouragement, and hopelessness—which can be alleviated by the reality of His Holy Presence.

Realizing your need for and asking for the Holy Spirit's presence within you is the first step to receiving His guidance. After all, how will you fulfill that need if you are unaware of the need for His Spirit and His guidance? A victim who chooses to allow Christ to lead and guide her life chooses an inspiring, purposeful, meaningful, fulfilling, hopeful life. Because that is what it means to be a Christian, a follower of Christ—and that is what it takes to become an *Overcomer* such as Christ. She can allow the darkness of abuse to die, and she can live again with a new life in Christ. When she gives permission for dark abuse thoughts to guide her mind, she can assume that, whatever she's worried about, that satan's got it. But, when she turns to the Light of hopeful possibilities to be set free from her abuse, she can be certain that God's got it!

A victim's past is in need of Spiritual healing along with a renewing of the mind and body. When a victim learns that, after accepting Christ the Holy Spirit dwells in her; she is able to draw power and wisdom from the *Spirit* within her. She begins to understand many new in-depth aspects of her life. "That your faith should not be in the wisdom of men but in the power of God" (1 Corinthians 2:5). For the first time, the victim begins to recognize, see, and hear *deep* things in her life that she was not aware of before (no matter her age). "But as it is written: 'Eye has not seen, nor ear heard, Nor have entered into the heart of man The things which God has prepared for those who love Him.' But God has revealed *them* to us through His Spirit. For the Spirit searches all things, yes, the deep things of God" (1Corinthians 2:9-10). There is a difference between a victim and an *Overcomer*: an *Overcomer* is sensitive to the stirrings of the Holy Spirit and therefore faces her present and future with faith and hope. Accept and add the tender touch of the Holy Spirit to your life—you will feel the positive difference in balancing your daily living!

For some people, the whole *idea* of being "born again" is very weird and even creepy, but it's only odd to those that don't understand the things of God. Those who are unable to comprehend and discern spiritual things generally criticize and sometimes persecute believers (born again Christians). This reaction is not uncommon. Jesus was persecuted for being a believer as well—so much so that He was hung on a cross for His belief in God the Father. It's not uncommon for agnostics or atheists to bully born-again Christians and say, "Well, if Jesus is alive, why don't you just have Him come back to Earth right now?" These nonbelievers have not read the gospel and God's plan for Jesus to return after *all* of His revelation has been completed. They don't comprehend the magnitude of His love for them, that He's even waiting for as many as will accept salvation so that none should perish! "The Lord is not slack concerning *His* promise, as some count slackness, but is longsuffering toward us, not willing that any should perish but that all should come to repentance"

(2 Peter 3:9). God's Word says that He is *love* and He will keep His Word and demonstrate that love even for nonbelievers; If God did not exist, we would not know or have *love*.

The discomfort that we suffer from unbelievers is all a part of being set apart from the world based on our Christian principles. However, there is an estimated over two billion Christians in the world that outnumber those that are determined to be agnostic or atheist persecutors. We can find God's love and encouragement through our brothers and sisters in Christ that are likeminded. Those that persecute Christians are not spiritually discerning, and this sadly prevents them from comprehending the Word of God and the *truth* about Christ—and the *freedom* and *peace* that He alone can give. Our role as Christians is not to be condemning, as they sometimes are to us, but to model the unconditional love and grace that Christ demonstrates to us daily. The following are some Scriptures with God's promises to send you the Holy Spirit as your Guide—your helper!

> "And when He has come, He will convict the world of sin, and of righteousness, and of judgment. However, when He, the Spirit of truth, has come, He will guide you into all truth, for He will not speak on His own *authority*, but whatever He hears He will speak; and He will tell you things to come" (John 16:8, 13).

> "But you shall receive power when the Holy Spirit has come upon you" (Acts 1:8).

> "But the Helper, the Holy Spirit, whom the Father will send in My name, He will teach you all things, and bring to your remembrance all things, that I said to you" (John 14:26).

> "And I will pray the Father, and He will give you another Helper, that He may abide with you forever--" (John 14:16).

> "Now hope does not disappoint, because the love of God has been poured out in our hearts by the Holy Spirit who was given to us" (Romans 5:5).

How does a victim of abuse become born of God (Spiritually born again)? In the same way that any person in this world does: the instructions are found in the Word of God. A person is born again by the Word of God; God the Father, Son, and Holy Spirit *are* the Word of God.

> "In the beginning was the Word, and the Word was with God, and the Word was God. And the Word became flesh and dwelt among us, and we beheld His glory, the glory as of the only begotten of the Father, full of grace and truth" (John 1:1, 14).

God's Word tells us that in order to be born of God and have eternal life (to be saved), we must repent of our sins and believe the Gospel, that Christ died for our sins, that He was buried, and that He rose again the third day after His death. Therefore, if you believe that Jesus is the Christ, our Savior, Who died for our sins and was buried and rose for the forgiveness of our sins, then you have made your home in heaven by believing in Him. It is *not* about making major positive changes in your life. You can make all of the changes necessary to improve your life and yet never truly believe the Gospel—consequently, never be saved. It's all about *faith!* If you are a believer, you are *then* ready to ask Him (the Holy Spirit) to come into your heart, and you will at that point become a born-again child of God.

> "For God so loved the world that He gave His only begotten Son, that whoever believes in Him should not perish but have everlasting life. For God did not send His Son into the world to condemn the world, but that the world through Him might be saved" (John 3:16-17).

Being born of God (born again) and being saved (salvation) go hand-in-hand, just like believing in the Christ and repentance of your sins go hand-in-hand. Once a person believes in Jesus, the person repents and experiences forgiveness.

> "To Him all the prophets witness that, through His name, whoever believes in Him will receive remission of sins" (Acts 10:43).

> "Most assuredly, I say to you, he who believes in Me has everlasting life" (John 6:47).

There is no specific day and right place or time that's perfect to ask Christ into your heart. *Any* day, time, or place is right to accept Christ—God. All you need to do is to feel led by the Spirit of God. Are you ready to ask Christ—the Holy Spirit—to dwell in you? To be born of God (born again)? "For as many as are led by the Spirit of God, these are sons of God" (Romans 8:14). Accept the challenge; through the Holy Spirit, you will have the *power* to overcome! Some people struggle with the issue of asking for forgiveness of their sins because they declare that they are good people and have led a life of good character and of good deeds, so *why* do they have to ask for forgiveness; can't they just state that they believe in Christ? It's not possible to believe in Christ without acknowledging that we sinned against Him and led Him to the cross. We were born in sin (through Adam and Eve); that's why He died—because of our sins. We are no different in our inborn sinful nature than the people in biblical times. We are *all* sinners by inheritance; we *need* to ask to be forgiven in order to reconcile and get right with God.

> "Even the righteousness of God, through faith in Jesus Christ, to all and on all who believe. For there is no difference; for all have sinned and fall short of the glory of God" (Romans 3:22-23).

This is why when you are ready to call upon Him to receive Christ (the Holy Spirit) and be born of God, you will have to pray a sinner's prayer. Everyone has a free ticket to heaven offered to them by God, waiting to be used. Now, again, this is totally optional; salvation and being born again is a very personal decision for a very personal relationship with God. As was stated earlier, He does give you your very own free will to choose and to make decisions about your life. Accepting salvation and the Holy Spirit is a condition of the heart. It is about your will; your mouth *cannot* pray and confess something you are *not* willing to do.

> "That if you confess with your mouth the Lord Jesus and believe in your heart that God has raised Him from the dead, you will be saved. For with the heart one believes unto righteousness, and with the mouth confession is made unto salvation" (Romans 10:9-10).

> "For 'whoever calls upon the name of the Lord shall be saved'" (Romans 10:13).

So you see, the miracle of life is not just at birth when your Creator formed you. "For You have formed my inward parts; You have covered me in my mother's womb" (Psalm 139:13). There's another miracle birth awaiting *you* whenever you're prepared to be born again. Are you feeling overwhelmingly fearful and confused? If so, Jesus (God's Son) wants to have a little visit with you. This may be an unforecasted meeting for you. However, today and the rest of your life can be mostly cloudy with a chance of nothing, or it can be a Son-shine day! If at any point as a victim of abuse, you are ready to receive Christ and be born of God, and would like to begin your journey as an *Overcomer* with your Heavenly Father as your Guide, you may want to pray something similar to this:

> *Father God, for reasons known to You, I am in need of Your forgiveness. I come to You today, asking for Your forgiveness for the life that I have lived and ask for Your forgiveness for_____. I believe that Your Son, Jesus Christ, died for my sins so that I could have eternal life. I now accept You, Jesus Christ, as my Lord and personal Savior, and I thank You for my gift of eternal life. Jesus, come into my heart; take charge, and transform me so that I may glorify and honor You with my life. I pray and ask for Your healing in the Name and power of Jesus, Amen.*

If you've just prayed that prayer and asked to receive Christ in your life, feel free to celebrate! Call out to Him; He's ready to listen. He's your new friend! Through the Holy Spirit, He's your new Companion. Visualize shaking His Hand and embrace the comfort of His long, outstretched Arms around you from now on and for all of your days. Feel free to break into a little dance—just about now, go ahead; there's no rule that says you can't dance. Even biblical people danced when they were overcome with joy—go for it! If dancing is not for you, sing a familiar tune to one of your favorite worship songs; sing out loud at the top of your lungs and *feel the joy*! Receiving Christ's Spirit in one's heart brings on an inexplicable, natural, ebullient mood! What if you feel *nothing*? That's okay, too. It could be like it is on your birthday; you feel nothing different in your body, but yet chronologically, something has changed. Today is your spiritual birthday—rejoice! And, while you're at it, begin praying for your unsaved loved ones; pray that God would send a spiritual laborer to minister to them and that they too would accept Christ. Go drench yourself in His Word. As you proceed in your new life in Christ, prepare yourself for your *Overcomer* divine battle!

Spiritual victory for a victim can only come as a result of being prepared for her *battle*. "The night is far spent, the day is at hand. Therefore let us cast off the works of darkness, and let us put on the armor of light" (Romans 13:12). "Put on the whole armor of God, that you may be able to stand against the wiles of the devil" (Ephesians 6:11). Your former armor may have included worry. To be girded with tools that include worry is to remain in despair. Put on His armor *now*. Part of His armor includes listening for His voice. Reading or listening to His Word via media will not only equip you with your directions for the day, weeks, and months to come, but it will inject a daily dosage of His love, strength, and power! This is not the end of your story, daughter of King Jesus; wear His armor and instead of remaining as a victim, be a warrior of His Kingdom!

This armor will protect you so that when you tune Him in, even while you're in the presence of a crowd with opinions and temptations, His voice is the only One that you choose to recognize and follow. Leave your irreversible past in His Hands and launch your new irrepressible life in Him as an *Overcomer*. The abuser's cunning, sly methods cannot penetrate a victim's spirit when she makes the Holy Spirit's warnings her daily concern. The abuser and his followers are like satan, just a sham! During those times when the abuser's or others' voices instill guilt in you for wanting out of the abuse, or satan whispers that you should stay and give the abuser just one more chance, ask Christ for strength beyond Eve so that you will not be cunningly deceived by the serpent himself, like when he led Eve's mind astray.

We discussed how Eve was deceived by satan and thus sin entered the world through his tempting of both Adam and Eve. The great news is that because Christ died for our sins, we no longer have to continue to inherit their disobedience and sin; we can choose obedience to God's commandments and His will for our lives. We can ask for His forgiveness if we ever slip into sin. We can choose Christ's obedient, sinless nature! Ask for the divine insight that Christ had when He knew satan was attempting to deceive Him; instead, He stood up to him with Truth (God's Word) and told him to go away: *"Away with you, satan!"* (Matthew 4:10). satan would love for you to identify yourself as a victim and stay a victim. An *Overcomer* is who you are; listen to satan no more!

God provides wisdom and discernment; satan provides only lies about you. satan would like you to believe that you are a victim by confusing your identity (*who* God created you to be) with your problem (victimization). You are not your problem (victim). You are a separate being; You are *not* identical to your problem—that is satan's lie. The truth of *who* you truly are is known and revealed by God Who created your *identity*. When the abuser stripped you of your identity, not only did he snatch your Earthly identity, but he also confiscated your identity in

Christ which you were given the day that you were born. satan knows your identity is in Christ, and like the abuser, he wants to steal it.

However, the Holy Spirit lives within you and knows the Truth about your identity. This is the same identity that Paul talks about in Philippians 1:6, "being confident of this very thing, that He who has begun a good work in you will complete *it* until the day of Jesus Christ." The *work* Paul is referring to is the *process* of us growing from salvation to becoming more like Christ until we go home to be with Christ or upon His return (whichever comes first). Have you ever heard someone say the person that they're in love with completes them? Or they introduce their spouse as their *other* or *better half*? That's like saying the other person completes their identity. God's Word tells us that Christ is the only One Who has the power to *create* and *complete* our *identity* throughout our lifespan (Colossians 2:8-10).

The Holy Spirit is *Truth* that you can count on: "I am the way, the truth, and the life" (John 14:6). satan slithers and is slathered with the untruth; he wants you to listen to him instead of Jesus, Who has already told you that *He* is the Truth and the Way and that His desire is for you to live life fully and in peace. When we're obedient to God's will for our lives, satan loses his power to tempt us. Listening to satan's deceptive talk about marriage and abuse is like sitting on his lap, hearing, and accepting his counseling lies. As an *Overcomer*, you will live to tell about satan's taunting demise on your broken victim life. God is ready for you to tell about your miraculous and wholesome healing. That is how God wants your story to end.

In the same way that our body requires daily nutritious food to be healthy, our Spirit and Mind have to have sound thinking as *daily* input in order to function properly. You are an *Overcomer!* Within you, you have been equipped with wise decision-making abilities. Even if you can only imagine barely surviving, stay with me here. Ask Him to redeem all of your confusion and to bring *peace* into your life that has been so out-of-control. Ask for the healing and health that only He can give. In order to change her outlook, a victim must change how she feels and sees herself—by adjusting her thinking as an *Overcomer*. A victim thinks about survival; an *Overcomer* seeks and obtains self-preservation. Whatever you feel, think, and do daily is who you become—become an *Overcomer*!

Go forward, His beloved, and become an *Overcomer* because you can't go wrong in that decision. His fathomless love and undefeated power will place you on the heights of an *Overcomer* life. No more loss of hope through your despair; instead He will wipe away your pain-filled tears and replace them with tears of joy. Your heart will overflow with His presence, replacing your victim annihilation with His power to create a new life in you. Christ was sent to create your life, not to destroy it. His illimitable power and strength can be at work within you—He gives you that gift. He promises to both provide His power and to protect you. And He's a promise-keeper!

The Bible prescribes and describes the wearing of God's armor as a power to fend off evil: "Therefore take up the whole armor of God, that you may be able to withstand in the evil day, and having done all, to stand. Stand therefore, having girded your waist with truth, having put on the breastplate of righteousness, and having shod your feet with the preparation of the gospel of peace; above all, taking the shield of faith with which you will be able to quench all the fiery darts of the wicked one. And take the helmet of salvation, and the sword of the Spirit, which is the word of God" (Ephesians 6:13-17).

If you're of a personality that enjoys putting fun and playfulness into your day, visualize yourself wearing your armor as if you're decked out looking like a powerful warrior! Hear the sounds of your armor clanking swiftly as you enter a room. If you prefer a change of attire for the day, be empowered emotionally and feel spiritually stronger by picturing yourself walking into the grocery store (or wherever) wearing your purple, royal cape and your crown as the daughter of a King. Refrain from the temptation of seeing yourself or placing yourself in the position of a victim. The Bible says that someday when the Lord your King calls you heavenward, He will gift you with the crown of life. "Blessed *is* the man who endures temptation; for when he has been approved, he will receive the crown of life which the Lord has promised to those who love Him" (James 1:12). For now, wear your proper Earthly crown as His princess. Go ahead—visualize yourself wearing your bejeweled crown! There are powerful Scriptural affirmations that a victim as an aspiring *Overcomer* can visualize and use. Affirmative visualizations can not only inspire one to be spiritually uplifted, but they can also result in one standing confidently. He offers you His Holy peaceful countenance. Accept it—own it—wear it!

Solution and healing from abuse don't come from human intelligence; they come from God's infinite love and wisdom. Your healing from abuse trauma will come from God and His Holy Spirit alone. Healing from abuse is one of God's Kingdom acts! Think about the disciples and the choices that they made—the life that they led *before* they received the Holy Spirit on Pentecost (Acts 2). It was the indwelling of the Holy Spirit that transformed and changed each disciple; they were not able to accomplish such change on their own. The *same* opportunity is offered to you. "Then Peter said to them, Repent, and let every one of you be baptized in the name of Jesus Christ for the remission of sins; and you shall receive the gift of the Holy Spirit. For the promise is to you and to your children, and to all who are afar off, as many as the Lord our God will call" (Acts 2:38-39). Since the gift and power of the Holy Spirit is invisible and cannot be scientifically measured within an individual's heart, it can remain unrecognized and more often than not, the victim is unaware of the valuable, infinite spiritual reserve that is at her disposal.

My focus when working with a victim is *not* just on the condition of her Spirit; it is balanced in evaluating the state of her Mind and Body. The goal is to help her obtain maximum improvement in order to heal her spiritually, mentally, and physically. Spiritual growth, mental awareness (brain education), nutrition, vitamin supplementation, exercise, insight-gaining, and changing a lifestyle of maladaptive habit toxins (body actions/behaviors) *all* become a part of the treatment plan. If the Spirit is aligned in equilibrium with the Mind and Body, there is an increased chance that a person will be able to experience and maintain harmony with their spiritual, emotional, and physical health. This balance can be obtained through Spiritual activities that feed the Spirit spiritual food: reading the Bible, devotionals, inspirational books or media, praying, and attending worship and fellowship events. The Spirit can act as a helper, comforter, and encourager and can uplift sufficiently for a person to access *peace* in the midst of extreme circumstances. This can be achieved by praying or connecting with others that can mentor and provide support spiritually.

Prayer is an important part of our relationship with the Spirit (God) within us. Prayer provides hope; prayer and hope go hand-in-hand—they are both as essential as breathing. The veracity of God's Word is that *all* Scripture is God-breathed (2 Timothy 3:16). If we skip His Word and praying to Him, we miss the portion of *His* breathing hope into us. When we lose His hope, our prayer and/or devotional time stops breathing and disappears along with that hope. Once the Holy Spirit has taken residence, it becomes a part of our vitals—a part of our life-giving bodily organs: the brain, lungs, heart, liver, and stomach. Prayer is the natural blood flow that is needed to keep your Spirit activated in your heart. Prayer is a source of life. It is like our breathing;

we wouldn't dream of stopping our ongoing breathing. Prayer provides vigor. That daily intimate communion, fellowship, and dialogue with God is of critical priority. Prayer is as essential to our vitality in life as our body is in producing, taking in, and maintaining its vital fluids! There's a truism that states, "Seven days without prayer makes one weak."

When the Holy Spirit is on active duty, prayer is not looked upon as a boring ritual but as more of a hunger for speaking with God and hearing from Him; we look forward to it like when we nourish ourselves with daily food intake. Our prayer time with God should be watched closely like when we read Nutrition Facts labels to check the Percent Daily Value of a food product! Consider incorporating the practice of using a Prayer Percent Daily Value as your guide to determine if you're getting sufficient spiritual nutrients in your Spirit, Mind, and Body. Are you low or balanced on spiritual nutrients? Note that the Food and Prayer Administration has not yet set a Daily Value for sporadic crisis prayers, and health experts recommend avoiding ritualistic prayer marathons to lower your risk of cardiovascular attacks. Similarly, there is no established Daily Value for prayerlessness. Alright, enough with the joking around! Let us continue with our mission! The point is that adding prayer to your food intake increases your Spiritual Nutrition Value and fortifies your daily diet.

Prayer time will always nurture and strengthen your Spirit; it is a reprieve that you have at your discretion all the time, which will direct you to healthy coping skills. God does not expect you to lobby repetitive memorized ritualistic prayers to Him just as He doesn't expect you to eat the same food every day. Prayer isn't an exercise; it's simply talking to God and listening for what he has to say about every aspect of our life, and it can be as simple as praising Him daily for Who He is and thanking Him for all He has done and all that He will do! Prayer will grant you the ability to live in an atmosphere of peace while working on living an abuse-free life.

God does answer prayer. Notice that Jesus never spoke of unanswered prayer. On the contrary, Jesus said with certainty, "And whatever things you ask in prayer, believing, you will receive" (Matthew 21:22). Your rebuttal right now could be, "Well, He hasn't always answered my prayers." Oh yes, He has, each and every time! You may not have seen the immediate answer in the way your will would want it answered, but whatever and however it's answered, it is according to *His* will, our best interest, His purposes for our life and that of others. God answers prayer within His supernatural revelations and not through our methodical or logical thinking.

A prayerful, spiritually-enlightened person can better handle *whatever* comes their way. Once a person gets a taste of having His Spirit within, they find Him to be without equal! It is a life-changing encounter with God. "Now the Lord is the Spirit; and where the Spirit of the Lord *is*, there *is* liberty. But we all, with unveiled face, beholding as in a mirror the glory of the Lord, are being transformed into the same image from glory to glory, just as by the Spirit of the Lord" (2 Corinthians 3:17-18). God's *peace* can be obtained any time daily simply by calling out to Him in prayer. Nourishing the Spirit is a reciprocal process. We spiritually feed ourselves to grow; in the process, while we are *receiving* from God, we are *giving* Him back our reverence by taking care of our Spirit.

If our Spirit is acknowledged and *not* left untapped (if we choose *not* to be spiritually dead, *and* we take care of feeding our Spirit with spiritual food), *then* our Spirit will be a living guide full of joy and peace inside and out, while we work on balancing our Mind and Body. When the Spirit is being continually fed, it grows to not only focus on the self but to expand the Mind to become other-oriented, humble, and selfless in behavior. But again, this can only be accomplished when we decide not to be spiritually dead and when we choose to live optimally and completely through the Spirit. Once you have activated your Spirit, you will have access to a Spiritual adrenaline that will override your anxiety flight-or-freeze amygdaloidal tendencies.

If our mind is now filtering in peaceful thoughts through our Spirit, then we are empowered to take action and balance God, family, relationships, work life, and recreation. When the Mind has peace flowing through it in the midst of trials and tribulations, it is better able to process both the positive and negative events of our lives with healthy adaptive patterns of living (patience and healthy problem-solving skills). As the Spirit leads the way, the Mind is able to reflect on situations without impulsive reactivity; then the Mind is better able to use the Spirit to discern and comfort the self or others. Expressly, don't tend to compartmentalize everything you've learned about the Mind in your brain alone. *If* you allow it, you won't be able to help but make some level of connection to your Spirit; instead, you should begin to focus on how your Body operates as a balanced whole. That's what happens when you become intentional about balancing your person!

Still not convinced as to *why* God (the Spirit) needs to be involved in this process of establishing a holistic well-being? Granted, God's Word does encourage us to seek help from one another. It does say, "Two *are* better than one, Because they have a good reward for their labor. For if they fall, one will lift up his companion. But woe to him *who is* alone when he falls, For *he has* no one to help him up. Though one may be overpowered by another, two can withstand him. And a threefold cord is not quickly broken" (Ecclesiastes 4:9-10, 12). God does acknowledge that it is proper, it is expected, and that there is strength in seeking supportive help from others, but that does not mean that we don't need Him.

If we have supportive friends, family, and/or professionals, *why* do humans need divine help from God? The answer is simple; there are specific ways that the Spirit of God can help—through which humans *cannot* help. The obvious way is God's commitment to us—it *is* everlasting (eternal). At the end of the day, there is no human being that is available to help twenty-four hours, seven days a week, 365 days yearly. God our Protector does not slumber or sleep (Psalm 121:3-4). God is omnipotent, omniscient, and omnipresent. Do you know anyone in this world that would be able to offer you a relationship with those qualities? Not on your life! You'll find that God is matchless when you pursue help from humankind. All humans are feeble and fallible under a crisis state. When we turn to God, our most difficult life circumstances serve us to educate our faith and reliance upon Him. Humans are humans, and they are in just as much need of supportive help in balancing their Spirit, Mind, and Body as anyone else is.

Humans are just flesh, and flesh expires—the Spirit does not. If you set your life on living through the Holy Spirit, your life will be in safe Hands. So place your hand in the Hand of the One who will not just hold it but console it, protect it, and lead it to the path of peace and safety. Our human needs exceed what mankind can do for us. Our human support system is necessary and great here on Earth in the natural realm, but God is our Protector in the world through the unseen realm—the supernatural realm. Are you having trouble believing in the unseen supernatural realm? Pray for God to increase and develop your faith in the unseen Father, Son, and Holy Spirit. Pray that you would be willing to accept His guidance and protection over your abuse. Sometimes victims don't mean to, but they have tug-of-wars with God—thinking they can out-strength Him with their aim at ending their abuse on their own. Are you through having a victim tug-of-war with God?

If you are not captious or contentious with God, divine help is limitless—through the Holy Spirit. Our natural human ability and gifts are limited, no matter what our level of education and intellect may be. *If* we have accepted the Holy Spirit within us, the help and work of the Holy Spirit will be manifested in us. He will be with you to work out your abuse for the good of all involved. "And we know that all things work together for good to those who love God, to those who are the called according to *His* purpose" (Romans 8:28). He is your divine Co-Worker. God is able to see through what our support system is unable to see within our past, present, and future. I've never known any human being to be able to deliver this type of supernatural help, have you? So, with man's limitations, where does our true help come from? It comes from God! God's help is actually only a *prayer* away. The Bible says, "My help *comes* from the LORD, Who made heaven and earth" (Psalm 121:2); "God *is* our refuge and strength, A very present help in trouble. Be still, and know that I *am* God. The Lord of hosts *is* with us; The God of Jacob *is* our refuge" (Psalm 46:1, 10a, 11). He is your Helper that's forever with you—He is Your Helper and Shelter!

God's Word in the Psalms has been read by many of faith who seek His comfort, strength, and guidance. Still and all, some skeptics see the Psalms as meaningless, poetic song Scriptures (without a divine purpose for inspiring the soul). The Psalms are viewed by some as ordinary inspirational poetry and songs, not taking into account that the 150 Psalms in the Bible coincide with the five books of Moses (Genesis-Deuteronomy). The fact that the Psalms correspond with the five books of Moses is significant because anyone that knows the story of Moses knows that Moses was a man of boundless faith. God appeared to Moses, and his encounter with God involved trusting God when God called him to release the Israelites from captivity. Moses had to believe in faith and trust that God would help him to accomplish what He had called him to do! Let's take a look at Moses' experience—for he too had to operate as an *Overcomer*.

In order to help Moses to fulfill the task of freeing the Israelites from further oppression, God inflicted upon Egypt ten plagues (calamities). He did this to contrast His omnipotence as God with the impotence of the numerous gods that the Egyptians worshipped *and* in order to convince Pharaoh (King of Egypt) to release the abused Israelites from slavery. Pharaoh surrendered after the tenth plague, which then facilitated Moses to lead the exodus of the Israelites. Moses had to depend on God's help to accompany him daily throughout the devastation of both the Israelites and the Egyptians. Moses knew where his *help* came from! Moses had to believe in faith that God *is* an all-powerful God and that He would separate the Red sea into two halves as He said He would. Therefore, Moses could lead the Israelites to walk on dry ground while crossing the parted sea! Moses also had to believe that God would free the Israelites, whether while Moses was alive or after his death—that God would do what He said He would do! It was soon after this that Moses had to trust God *again* and solicit His help with the delivery of the Ten Commandments (which are still God's commandments today). Your *hope* in this season of your life as a victim is ultimately found in your willingness to *trust* God—as an *Overcomer*—like Moses did.

The *same* love and promises God made to Moses are available to you and me today. God never changes—He is immutable. So, claim His Scriptural promises! His Word is Truth that's unchangeable, and it is His Word that He will do. He promises that His Word can be counted on, "and being fully convinced that what He had promised He was also able to perform" (Romans 4:21). Base your foundation of hope on Jesus Christ's Word and unchanging nature. God loves His children whom He created with the same profound, unconditional love that He demonstrated to Moses and the Israelites. What parent loves one child more than the other? We love each one of our children equally in the same way that God does us. God loved our ancestors in biblical times the same way that He continues to love us and our descendants today: "For there is no partiality with God" (Romans 2:11). God's love and promises from biblical times remain the same today and all of our days because of His love and His deity. "For I *am* the LORD, I do not change" (Malachi 3:6); "'I am the Alpha and the Omega *the* Beginning and *the* End,' says the Lord, who is and who was and who is to come, the Almighty'" (Revelation 1:8); "Every good gift and every perfect gift is from above, and comes down from the Father of lights, with whom there is no variation or shadow of turning" (James 1:17).

The difficulty humans have believing in the deity of Christ and accepting help from God's divine intervention is usually related to pride and a a lack in faith—a lack of humility. In order to submit with faith, Moses had to humble himself unto God, something that was not difficult for him to do because he was already a humble man: "(Now the man Moses *was* very humble, more than all men who *were* on the face of the earth.)" (Numbers 12:3). Ask Christ to exterminate your pride and give you the fruit of humility. It's *not possible* for God to work with our Spirit and our life if we're unwilling to ask for help because our pride gets in the way. As an *Overcomer*, Moses' character was built on unwavering faith and prayerfulness; laying all of his problems and decisions before God and surrendering them to Him, he built up his courage to trust God to take charge in spite of his and others' painful circumstances. Moses *never* doubted that God would protect the Israelites through an exodus from abusive slavery and grant them their promised land! A victim can transmute her victimization into her own personal exodus to her promised land—as an *Overcomer*.

Moses put God first in his life—he was drawn out as one of God's humans called to serve Him because He believed in God's mighty power to help him with whatever he was called to do. Just as the Psalms irrevocably state that God is our Maker, Helper, and the Lord above and over all, so do the accounts of the books of Moses. The Psalmists and Moses were *Overcomers*. So, be like the Psalmists and Moses. Accept God's help *today*, and He will infill you with His Spirit! Just say it like Os Hillman: T.G.I.F (Today God Is First).

Balancing Your Mind
Let's talk about the Mind and its connection to the Spirit. Your Spirit plays a big part in developing and shaping your Mind. The Spirit helps the Mind take inventory of life situations, to explore one's will as well as the wisdom in how our decisions or choices impact ourselves and others in the present and future. Seeking God's help and His will for one's life—and His will for others—is a *mindfulness* decision. *Mindfulness* entails purposely paying attention to present experiences as they occur moment by moment without reacting with mindless thoughts or actions. *Mindless* thoughts or actions are symptoms of brokenness in the mind. Being actively *mindful* in all life activities is a power booster to the *neurotransmitters* in our brain. Something else to consider then, is your neurotransmitters. Neurotransmitters are chemical substances located and released in the brain. A neurotransmitter is produced and secreted by a neuron that then diffuses across a synapse, which causes excitation or inhibition of yet another neuron. A deficiency in these neurotransmitters can chemically imbalance your mood. (Neurotransmitters and mood affect are further discussed in the section on Balancing Your Body.)

Mindful behavior elevates your immune system and self-esteem, mediates your thoughts, moderates your appetite, regulates your stress levels, and develops your cognitive skills and peace of mind. This kind of *mindfulness* can ignite a human's awareness, which then enhances the sense of knowing and enables the person to further experience being fully awakened in the mind (fully alive), culminating in a new way of noticing details and obtaining a clarity and a sense of energy which then supports the person's Spirit, Mind, Body and overall social well-being.

Mindfulness-based behaviors are a vital part in the treatment of the whole person. It's not an activity in which you have to stop what you're doing; it's a natural mental process that can become a daily part of your functioning. Regardless of outward circumstances, a person's practice of *mindfulness* is associated with learning to approach their challenging circumstances rather than withdrawing from them. The research interprets this as a sign of *neural resilience*. *If* a person is *willing* to practice *mindfulness* consistently, *mindfulness* can train the Mind, and it can become a way of being which shapes the ongoing neurological health of the person's life.

This brings us to a discussion of the neurological aspects of the Mind—the brain. This is relevant to discuss because having knowledge of *how* our brain develops can remarkably change *how* we see things and *how* we respond or react to them. It's important to learn about our brain because neurological studies find that our life experiences *do* shape the structure of our brain. Scientific study has determined that our brain actually develops and changes throughout our lifespan and is indeed shaped by our genes and experience. This indicates that our brain has neuroplasticity, which gives our brain cells the ability to perceive, respond, and adapt flexibly. A dictionary definition of *plasticity* is "the capacity for continuous alteration of the neural pathways and synapses of the living brain and nervous system in response to experience or injury." Synapses allow information to travel from one neuron to another; when neurons communicate, they create neural pathways. Research shows that our brain continues to reorganize itself in order to maintain its optimal efficiency throughout our entire aging process. "The human brain remains open to changing in response to experience throughout the lifespan."[1] "Recent findings in the field of neuroplasticity reveal that the human brain remains open to changing in response to experience throughout the lifespan. It can grow new synaptic connections, make new myelin, and even grow new neurons from neural stem cells that develop into fully mature integrative neurons within several weeks."[2]

This is always exciting information for everyone to become aware of. It's helpful because if our brain continues to develop and take shape throughout our life, then this provides hope for those that are seeking to improve their state of Mind! This means that if we actively pursue changing our life experiences, then our brain (our mind) and our way of thinking (our perspective) throughout our life *can* change. Our brain's capacity to change is based on the fact that the brain is an organ that has neural *plasticity*. "Research suggests that there is far more plasticity in the adult brain than was previously believed possible, even in the face of neurological impairments."[3] YES! Can you get excited about the amazing fact that our brain is flexible and bendable like soft plastic? What this confirms is that once you begin to consistently work toward developing your brain, it's actually moldable like clay!

How can you make good use of your brain's capability to be shaped and changed? This is only possible through your extensive practice of using and balancing both the left and right hemispheres of your brain. This is called *brain integration*, integrating the left and the right brain when processing information and interacting with the self and others. Of course, in order for our brain to change, we have to be open and willing to learn, explore, and practice new ideas and new ways to operate. Changing the brain is an intentional process that requires focus and attention to our ways of thinking and behaving in the past, present, and anticipated future. To change our brain purposely, we must be willing to unlearn our old ways of thinking and doing. In order for the brain to change, we have to unlearn reactive interacting to circumstances with the self and others and instead learn to respond appropriately. The brain is able to change as you take care of it, not only through establishing healthy responses to circumstances and your social interaction with the self and others, but also through proper nutrition, sleep, and exercise.

Since *brain integration* is the key to developing and changing the brain, let's briefly review what the left and right hemispheres of the brain are responsible for. Our left brain is verbal and capable of learning multiple languages; it conducts our intellectual reasoning and logical thinking for us. Our right brain has the capability of observing and exhibiting non-verbal communication; it is creative, and it senses emotion and can store our autobiographical memory (our stories of what has happened in our life). Studies have demonstrated that when humans make limited use of only one side of the brain (either left or right) and both sides are not used in a balance, there's no brain integration of the two sides of the brain, and no brain integration leads to rigidity and reactive chaos. Acquiring brain integration therefore leads to developing good mental health. You can either do the research yourself on *how* to develop and integrate your brain or seek a professional to assist you in this process.

It is impossible for a victim's brain to go unchanged if she decides to become an *Overcomer*, because as was said earlier, we *can* change our brain neurologically with experiences. The victim's new experiences can facilitate brain changes into an *Overcomer* perspective. As an *Overcomer*, your new brain changes allow you to have a new brain appraisal center whereby you can incorporate what's old in your life or eliminate it according to your new standards and goals for mental well-being. In other words, brain integration allows a victim the freedom to either continue to live with emotionally volcanic outbursts and total meltdowns, where logic and reason don't operate (highly emotionally charged thought processes or interactions are right brain), *or* to learn to differentiate what's on a higher thinking plane (left brain) and link the right and left brain interactions in a balanced way. When a victim has only practiced using her right brain, whenever the abuser or someone who reminds her of the abuser approaches her, it's like someone has just called out to her, "satan's at the door!" Integration of the brain is a healthy state of mind; it's when the right and left brain work functionally as a whole which then results in mental health harmony.

You can develop your brain, and your Mind can be expanded through the use of resources, which fortify the areas of your life that you specifically need to grow in. Moreover, praying and nature can serve as additional resources to calm the mind; God's creation of a sunrise, horizon, and a sunset can nurture a person into thinking more deeply and peacefully. Simply spending fifteen minutes quietly reading the Bible and an inspirational devotional for the day can influence your entire mind and way of thinking! Some of my patients that are unable to sit down and have a quiet devotional time due to their circumstances usually multi-task and use their daily walk to pray and communicate with God. How does God come into the picture in the areas of the mind and brain? Neuroscientists, Andrew Newberg, M.D., Mark Robert Waldman and others have documented research findings that God can actually change your brain.

In their book "How God Changes Your Brain," Dr. Newberg and Mark Robert Waldman state:

> "Our research team at the University of Pennsylvania has consistently demonstrated that God is part of our consciousness and that the more you think about God, the more you will alter the neural circuitry in specific parts of your

brain. That is why I say, with the utmost confidence, that God can change your brain. Intense, long-term contemplation of God and other spiritual values appears to permanently change the structure of those parts of the brain that control our moods, give rise to our conscious notions of self, and shape our sensory perceptions of the world. The moment we encounter God, our brain begins to change. Only human beings can think themselves into happiness or despair, without any influence from the outside world. Thus, the more we engage in spiritual practices, the more control we gain over our body, mind, and fate."[4]

Your Spirit plays a big part in developing your brain and shaping your Mind. Balancing our Mind is indeed a conscientious effort that's worth the time and energy; it is rewarding in its results for the self and others! There is more to a person than simply an aligned *sense of being* through the Spirit, Mind, and Body. "You," the "unique you," are in the presence of your Spirit, Mind, and Body. No matter what horrendous life circumstance you're undergoing, *"you"* are *there!* While in the middle of working on balancing your Spirit, Mind, and Body, *you* become aware of *"you"* and *all* of your God-given talents (gifts) that are no one else's but *yours*. Your face and body looking different than everyone else's isn't sufficient evidence that you are *unique*. There are things that *you* alone are capable of accomplishing that others are not able to; *vice versa*, there are areas of knowledge in which others run circles around you. Sometimes in balancing the Spirit, Mind, and Body, people become aware of their awesome possibilities and what they can achieve, while others learn of their limitations. By the same token, a limitation can direct one to other options and even provide incentive for other options that don't have that limitation.

Becoming aware and seeing one's unique self, potential, and limitations can develop an appreciation for one's gifts, the gifts of others, and empathy for those that are limited in their gifts. One example the evidence that a person's Spirit is growing and *is* working in their lives is the obvious change in their unworried and gratified attitude with which they *now* carry themselves. There is a new appreciation for the grace of being alive and the option of obtaining a healthy life, for being allowed to call this wonderful world God created our temporary home. This calmness of Spirit then allows the person to not be so self-focused, and they can now extend themselves to rejoice and celebrate the gifts and blessings of others. Aligning the Spirit, Mind, and Body scales down one's actions from blaming or judging others for their limitations. Balancing and aligning the Spirit, Mind, and Body provides an opportunity to develop trust in oneself and others, to challenge the self to overcome one's own limitations! *If* your Spirit, Mind, and Body *are* balanced, you can identify your gifts more readily and are more willing to offer *your* gifts in service to others.

When a person openly and objectively works on aligning their Spirit, Mind, and Body, their brainpower is maximized. Positive brain synapses develop when you're experiencing the feel-good outcomes of re-aligning your Spirit, Mind, and Body. By the way, if during the process of intentionally balancing your Spirit, Mind, and Body, you notice yourself feeling exceptionally good, stop and deeply inhale to savor the moment and affix that experience. This will assist you in developing positive brain synapses more quickly (as positive information travels through the synapse, it signals feel-good neurotransmitters to be released). When you are aligned, you are able to make life decisions more efficiently; the Spirit opens up new pathways that allow your

Mind to be more flexible and at peace, and your Body is able to use the insight to fulfill the purpose for *your* unique *you*! You will always have your Spirit, Mind, and Body until death, but working on balancing them in a healthy way is pivotal as a life-and-death responsibility *if* you are going to respect God, yourself, and others.

Growing in Spirit as a victim only evolves *if* the person is willing to go to task for victory over abuse. A healed *Overcomer* life does not involve struggling for victory but rather believing in, claiming, and accepting the victory that has already been offered through Christ. Knowing Christ means knowing victory! When this divine *truth* settles in and dwells in your Spirit, your mind will no longer expect to be satan-defeated; you will not view yourself as a victim failure. Instead, you will receive the Holy Spirit's conviction that you can live a victorious *Overcomer* life! There are no limits to the good possibilities for your life when a Holy Spirit Mind is involved. Faith is not just about belief in Christ but also about what you are willing to allow Christ to do in you through the unmeasurable limitless power of the Holy Spirit. Once you allow the Spirit to work within you—your Mind and Body never have to go at it alone! Talk to God in prayer and have a devotional time with Him; He does hear you when you ask Him for guidance. When you speak to Him, listen for His voice through the Spirit; He will whisper words of comfort and implant wisdom in your mind in the midst of your chaos. Your only required step is to speak to Him and listen. Use your Holy Spirit-listening instinct and experience His voice in the stillness. Be like Samuel in the Bible; learn to discern God's voice through His Spirit in you and just say to Him, "Speak, for Your servant hears" (1 Samuel 3:10).

If you find it difficult to discipline yourself (to structure your devotional time with the Lord), try combining it with an activity that you routinely do, such as breakfast time. Breakfast is a daily nutrition process; the only time we don't have breakfast is when, as the word states, we break the fast (while we rest). That's the same pattern that our spiritual (quiet) time should have. Make it a fun time with Him—as you nourish your Body, you will feed your Spirit and Mind—*and* delight in the fact that you're having breakfast with your King! Having breakfast with the King of Kings will not only increase the meaningfulness of your morning meal, but it will fortify you with some Spiritual food. Besides your quiet devotional time, take additional time whenever you can to read His Word. God speaks to us through His Word; listen carefully. Whether you have trudged through the cycle of abuse for months or years, the Spirit (Holy Spirit) *is* your Global Positioning System (GPS). It's important to read God's Word, but it is most important to understand His message and directions from it. When, as a victim, you are at a fork in the road, it's time to pull over and come to a stop to consult the *way* the Lord would have you go. "There is a way *that seems* right to a man, But its end *is* the way of death" (Proverbs 16:25); "For the ways of the LORD *are* right" (Hosea 14:9). Don't forget to have your Bible with you at all times as it is your compass; it *is* your initial point (the fixed reference point). He is your Master Engineer!

If you follow God's Word and His instructions, you're sure to be heading in the precise direction of His purpose for your life. Balancing the Spirit, Mind, and Body is similar to a lifetime diet of healthy choices which can only begin with Spiritual nourishment—as more than just willpower is needed. There are choices that have to be made, and some choices have to be eliminated from your lifestyle diet. God's wisdom will sustain you on the road that is fruitful for you. The living Christ is ever-present in your heart now in good times and bad times. Be aware of His presence within you and walk with Him as He guides you through His wisdom and infinite companionship. God promises to make you fit and equipped for all that He calls you to do. In order to receive the wondrous and purposeful plan He has for you, you have to maintain an adventurous attitude toward Him at all times. Listen to what He requires of you, claim it, own it, and set Him alight as you walk through it. And, while you're reading His Word, ask Him which direction to go and at which landmark you should stop and settle because He knows the way! Go to Him with any concerns or questions; nothing is too small or too big for Him to handle. He's your Commander-in-Chief, and He will more than willingly lead the way and fight this battle with you!

Years ago, when doctors made house calls and one could indeed call the doctor and talk to him personally, they used to say as they handed you their prescription (Rx), "Take this and call me in the morning." It's no different nowadays; your Master Physician is saying today, "take this (His Word) and call me in the morning." Quiet Bible reading time is a daily Rx to an ongoing relationship with God and freedom from pain. Now that's a dose of good medicine! Christ comforts you through His Love and His Peace during and after your time of pain. Christ relieves and heals your pain. He restores you as you call upon Him "Because His compassions fail not. *They are* new every morning" (Lamentations 3:22-23).

Perhaps you may see prayer or devotional time as a rote experience, but once entering the spiritual realm of God's throne, there's a desire to return to that sacred place, not just during those crisis days, but also during quiet times or worship days as well. Prayer is not meant to be an empty, routine religious form; it should not feel like a repetitive ritual because through the Holy Spirit one continues to gain new wisdom from reading God's Word (even though God's Word remains the same). Reading God's Word expands our spirit. Converse with the Lord from the silence of your wounded heart; share the details of your agony. Sure, He already knows what you have been going through, and you may think it's such a bore to Him for you to spell out your worries when He's already aware, but He never pushes Himself on anyone and instructs us specifically to seek Him out, just as you would a friend. Honestly, you wouldn't feel as an imposition if you were calling on a friend to ventilate some of your anxieties and painful issues, would you?

If you haven't reached out to the Lord in a while, don't waste any time in self-reproach for not seeking Him first while you've been in pain. Instead, apologize for your absence from His presence, and immediately you will find His Grace and the strength of His renewed relationship with you because His immanent Spiritual presence has been right there all along. All you need is to be aware of a yearning in your deepest being for His total presence in your circumstances—and you will then feel His presence infusing into your hurting heart. Go ahead and re-commit yourself anew to Christ!

Yes, feeling His presence is unbelievable, and hearing His Spirit tenderly speaking to you through His Word, that feeling of His complete love, is indescribable! Prayer time is like allowing God to massage your heart. Sure, you can feel His unconditional love daily and at other times besides your prayer time, but spending time with Him in prayer increases your sense of His Presence and the feeling of His radical love and commitment to you. It also allows you the time and freedom to praise Him and to reciprocate and express your love for Him. Time in prayer and the development of your spiritual growth is an expression of your love and commitment to Him. Prayer is a mindful act of worship.

Reading God's Word doesn't just realign and balance your Spirit, Mind, and Body, but it also allows you to *listen* to His guidance, to make decisions on life-changing choices that you may have to make. Reading His Word enhances your Spiritual maturity. It's impossible to maintain complete fellowship with God and remain narrow-minded in Spirit. He is the way to spiritual maturity and the road toward the Spirit, Mind, and Body living an abundant life. This consulting with God and the Holy Spirit can become a matter of releasing bad choices and cultivating good choices. As a victim, you may have to disown bad choices in order to develop the good choices. This means casting bad choices out of your life and never allowing for their return.

Those that implement the wisdom gained from God's Word and balance the Spirit, Mind, and Body are the ones that mature and embrace the discipline of seeking a healthy relationship with the self and others. In particular, they have learned to seek *peace* at all divine costs. This pursuit of *peace* does not mean the victim has to avoid *all* conflict in relationships at any price. It doesn't mean that the victim has to force herself to reconcile with unhealthy relationships. A victim *can* heal without reconciling with toxic relationships through the forgiveness of the self and others. This means that the victim has already done *everything* under the guidance of her Heavenly Father to work through the intense conflicts peacefully (with the intention that these relationships could be restored, strengthened, and sustained), and in some cases this effort has not been reciprocated.

God knows when we have Spiritually and Mindfully done our very best to strive to preserve harmony and righteousness in our relationships. We can count on His help and direction when others don't cooperate to sustain a healthy relationship with us. God cares right down to the very last detail of your suffering. "Indeed we count them blessed who endure. You have heard of the perseverance of Job and seen the end *intended by* the Lord—that the Lord is very compassionate and merciful" (James 5:11). "Is anyone among you suffering? Let him pray" (James 5:13). Long-suffering in an abusive relationship is filled with signs that point to your Creator as your *only* and final destination for guidance.

The very first relationship to strive to preserve is our relationship with God—the balancing of the rest of our relationships then follows through Him. As humans, *if* our Spirit is nourished to its highest potential, *and* our Mind and Body are taken care of optimally, then we can accomplish the balancing of Spirit, Mind, and Body and reap the flow of Spiritual *peace*. Aligning *your* relationship with God and *all* of your relationships through His Spirit is to your advantage. Aligning your Spirit with God leads to the balancing of your Mind and Body that then brings on personal, Spiritual healing *and* the healing of past relationships, which *can* have profound life-changing affects for yourself, your loved ones, and even the world that you live in. Some of the noticeable signs that you are aligning and balancing your Spirit with your Mind and Body are the following: letting go of your fear, focusing on the positive, and uncannily deciphering when *yellow flags* and *red flags* are approaching.

> "'For 'who has known the mind of the LORD that he may instruct Him?' But we have the mind of Christ" (1 Corinthians 2:16).

> "For God has not given us a spirit of fear, but of power and of love and of a sound mind" (2 Timothy 1:7).

> "Finally, brethren, whatever things are true, whatever things *are* noble, whatever things *are* just, whatever things *are* pure, whatever things *are* lovely, whatever things *are* of good report, if *there is* any virtue and if *there is* anything praiseworthy—meditate on these things" (Philippians 4:8).

One of the challenges that an *Overcomer* has to deal with (which, for some victims, is one of the reasons they decide not to leave the abusive relationship) is the *fear* in their mind of having lost months or years of their life and not being able to have the opportunities they had prior to the abusive relationship. It's such a prevalent issue in the mind of most victims that it warrants a discussion on how to deal with this common concern. Many victims convert lost time in the abusive relationship into a future with limitations. The *Overcomer* needs to *not* worry about lost time and should instead go forward with no regrets and a vision of faith for a safe life in her future. Having put your safety and the safety of your children into perspective, knowing that the choice of not leaving would have set off the boomerang effect on you and your children is of help—know that you made the healthy decision no matter how much time was lost.

In Joel 2:25-26, God promises that He will *restore* to you the years of your suffering where much was taken from you, and He reassures you that you will be satisfied, that He will deal with you wondrously, and that you shall never again be put to shame. I have watched hundreds of former victims that feared and viewed the loss of time as a handicap to their future, but they have indeed seen this Scriptural promise fulfilled in their lives. The reason this promise being fulfilled becomes so evident in an *Overcomer*'s life is because God shows up whenever one of His children calls on His Name, and He *does* what He says in His Word. He, unlike others, never forgets about you. If you have asked Him to restore the years you lost during the abusive relationship, He is a God of second chances! Yep, He does do-overs. He will restore the years that the abuser stole from you! We serve a God that rises above time and space. Since God is not a God of mediocrity, He *will* make up for all of that lost time and then some. He will restore the lost time that you're worried will keep you from reaching the goals that you had to forego while in abusive captivity.

God's in charge of time in our universe—not the abuser. You may be tempted to think that because you decided to stay and try to work things out, fruitlessly, that this means that it's impossible for you to retrieve all of the missed opportunities in your life because you spent that time working on the abusive marriage. God's mind doesn't think or operate in that way; He is willing and able to turn back the hands of time for anyone that turns to Him with their needs and dreams. If your goals and dreams are in line with God's plans for the purpose(s) in your life, God will arrange for you to make up for that lost time.

God *loves* you. He is a redeeming God; He is willing to turn the clock back or forward and do *whatever* is necessary to heal wrong choices or deliver productive time. The Holy Spirit is your helper to do *whatever* is right the next time around. Isaiah 38:7-8 depicts the experience of King Hezekiah when he was very ill. His response to his terminal illness was to cry out to the Lord, and he asked for restoration and healing. God answered this prayer and not only healed him, but also sent a message to him through Isaiah that He was going to add fifteen more years to Hezekiah's life. When Hezekiah heard the excellent news, he wanted a sign from God indicating that he was healed, so he asked God to show a sign by lengthening that day, and God did (by approximately ten hours)! If God moved the clock back and forward for Hezekiah, don't you think He can do the same for you?

God is always more than willing to restore what the enemy steals from you. So, the good news is that you have *not* missed *any* opportunities of which God is not aware, and He *can* bring back any past opportunity or even better ones that will fulfill the remainder of your life. Age is not a qualifying criteria for any missed goals that you may have had, and even if there was a career goal that had an age limit, you can rest assured without a shadow of a doubt that if God had that career goal in mind for you, *He* has the power to have made it come into fruition in spite of the abuser being in your life. God doesn't need our supervision to direct Him as to in what order our career moves should go in. He is God. God is quite aware of the time that you invested in a relationship that made time stand still. He *can* recoup and restore all of those months or years that you regret not applying to your personal goals. That is the divine mindset of God about time. That is the way an *Overcomer* mind thinks.

God's love and favor allow you to take that time you feel you wasted and make up for it. All He has to have is your commitment to Him in your new life, your request for restoration of time, and He *will* transform your former years of abuse into rewarding opportunities for the blessings toward the latter years of your life. As a victim, your mind can choose to dwell on the lost time, but that would only feed into a defeated victim mentality. An *Overcomer's* bold mindset believes in faith, that there's *nothing* that she and God can't accomplish together—including making up for lost time. Victims give up readily their goals and dreams which only empowers the abuser that much more. It's time to end your slavery to all of the oppressive documents that you have been storing and saving in your victim mind data files. Press delete and begin to key in and save your mindful thinking *Overcomer* data!

Yes, it's unfair that you sacrificed months, years, or your entire life for this abusive relationship. However, focusing on the unchangeable and permanent loss of time is *not* going to restore those years for you. It is your faith and commitment as an *Overcomer* that will exchange the loss of time for an *even better* Spirit, Mind, and Body. That is the type of mindset that will restore and resolve your future. God's plan for your life is not for you to settle for a high-handed, autocratic lifestyle under the dictatorship of your abuser's way of thinking. Your abuser's mind thinks that your life is over and that you can't regain the good in life that God means for you to have. Does your Mind want to think like the abuser or like an *Overcomer*? *Overcomers* think and develop a keener appreciation of the depth of God's plan for their lives and now notice the world which He created and His plan for it. Start now; ask Him to jump-start your energy in order to restore your freedom from abuse. Ask to be re-charged and healed permanently within your Spirit, Mind, and Body.

Nothing is inexecutable with God. He can change what was meant to harm you in past times into productive present and future years. So reach out to Him right *now*, ask Him to give you another chance at life. All that's required on your part when you ask Him to restore your past years is that you pray and believe in faith that God will follow through, that you will be victoriously triumphant no matter how severe your prior abusive circumstances were. Some victim's minds won't allow God to intervene. They have shared with me that they think they have messed up their lives with making so many wrong choices; they say that they just know God won't help them out anymore! God, our God, is a God of justice (See Isaiah 30:18). Your abuser and others may have neglected and abused you, but God knows your individual case—and your plea. He promises He will make things right for you as your Advocate. He will have mercy upon you and will step in and act on your behalf. God will take your case into His Hands *now* as you pray to forgive yourself and the abuser(s), and He will honor your request for a renewed mind and an *Overcomer* life. You will never experience a renewed mind if you don't ask Him for it. God has the power to bring about your renewal if you permit His divine intervention. After all, He is not called "Wonderful Counselor" (Isaiah 9:6) for no reason. Your long-term abuse is real—but so is God.

God is totally aware of all of your abusive incidents. For every one of your plaintive cries as a victim, God's character as your Counselor will show up! He will see to it that *justice* is served in your case. Have you ever observed a fiery trial either in person or via media? Those prosecuting attorneys don't peter out. Imagine having a *divine* Counselor that performs miracles and never tires out, and imagine what *He* can do in your defense! God *understands*. You have already experienced His miracles because He has been performing a miracle in your heart every time you experience His peace while undergoing unbearable suffering! His advocacy and understanding of your case is limitless. "Have you not known? Have you not heard? The everlasting God, the Lord, The Creator of the ends of the earth, Neither faints nor is weary. His understanding is unsearchable" (Isaiah 40:28).

If the judicial system does not give you the justice that you deserve, God will see to it as your vindicator that you no longer remain oppressed. As the Creator of our universe, He has the power to deal with the abuser Himself one-on-one. *Trust* Him as your Counselor to settle your case with the abuser once and for all. Trust God to be thorough in His judgment of righteousness. It's time for you to move up to the level of an *Overcomer*! "For we know Him who said, 'Vengeance is Mine, I will repay,' says the Lord. And again, 'The Lord will judge His people'" (Hebrews 10:30).

I realize that it's easier to be complacent or give up those former years and not start over to pursue your goals or dreams. However, with that mindset you will have to live with the regret(s) of "what if" and what could have been if you had only entrusted your present and your future to God. Don't allow your mind to store apathy, discouragement, negative thinking, or the thinking of others to mobilize your thoughts or actions. If you want to think like and be an *Overcomer,* use your positive thoughts and self-talk to nutritiously nourish and nurture your mind just like you use food to nourish your body. The Bible contains Scriptures that admonish us to stop thinking about or doing an unproductive activity/action/behavior and to start replacing/substituting it with a productive one. When an unproductive behavior is stopped without replacing it with a renewed productive behavior, it leaves room for returning back to the destructive habitual pattern of thinking and doing.

Break away from old victim patterns before they break you by developing and putting into action the replaced *Overcomer* principles! Make living an abuse-free life filled with *Overcomer* principles a daily practice. An *Overcomer* lives out what she has learned and thus she begins her voyage into peace. It's easier to nurture the ideal of becoming an *Overcomer* than to apply it and live it out. You essentially have a mind-fill, don't ignore it or dump negativity into it. Do not listen to yourself or others say negative things about you, whether out loud or in your mind. Don't allow others to run your mind for you. Stop right now—do not say negative things about yourself. "And my speech and my preaching *were* not with persuasive words of human wisdom, but in demonstration of the Spirit and of power, that your faith should not be in the wisdom of men but in the power of God" (1 Corinthians 2:4-5). Prepare your Spirit, Mind, and Body *daily* to declare that even though you've lost all hope to make up for lost time you're going to stand *strong* in faith on *all* of the promises that God has made to you regarding His love, ability, and power to restore you.

Trust in what God has in mind for you. As your Promise-Keeper, He gives you His Word that His plans are not to harm you but to give you hope and a future: *Believe* that He *can* provide you with a prosperous future. "For I know the thoughts that I think toward you, says the LORD, thoughts of peace and not of evil, to give you a future and a hope. Then you will call upon Me and go and pray to Me, and I will listen to you. And you will seek Me and find *Me,* when you search for Me with all your heart" (Jeremiah 29:11-13).

This is a critical time of decision for you. How is *your* mind going to think? I am talking about deciding how your mind as an *Overcomer* thinks now. This can either be a breaking point or a breakthrough for your divine destiny. Becoming an *Overcomer* requires a counter transformation from victim thinking. That is why you must maintain God's Word as the forefront of your foundation of strength. Keep your *Overcomer* vision on the forefront of your Spirit *and* Mind as opposed to the victim's "give up" and "what's the use?" attitude. Stand *strong* in the ground that you've gained thus far. Do not listen to the voices of the abuser and others that don't see you as God sees you. That is satan speaking and undermining your strength. Refuse to let your victimization define or defeat you. Choose not to look at your past victim role as a setback in your life but as an *Overcomer* comeback! Don't lose your focus on the future as an *Overcomer*—stay the course. Do not step back into your hopeless mindset. God has promised to vindicate you!

No trauma is so hopeless that one has to give in to it. When we do that, we undermine the grace, mercy, and power of our Savior. Christian faith is not the same as being an optimist. It is thinking about and knowing that even at one's most vulnerable, wounded state of need, there is hope because God's presence is there, and He has promised to come to one's aid in times of trouble. Believe and persevere even though you don't see immediate signs of change. Don't give in to satan, who only wants your mind to be lackluster and slow in faith. Instead, buckle up and hold on to your seatbelt of fast-paced *faith* because you serve a God that is the Creator of both your mind *and* time! You can trust Him. He will in *His time* accomplish all that He has purposed for your life. Expect that *if* you call out to God—He's going to *show up* to *help you*. He's a twenty-four-seven God. His sustaining power never fails. Oh, what a God you have! Give your Savior a shout-out!

Once upon a time while I was in Basic Combat Training, I noticed that my drill sergeant (the one who got in my face daily and yelled at me in the loudest voice I had ever heard) was in front of me walking backward and another drill sergeant (who was drill sergeant of the quarter) was walking alongside of me. Both were giving me the evil eye of contempt, just waiting for me to make a wrong move! For whatever reason, I was the only one assigned two drill sergeants to attempt to break me into weakness and giving up. That is exactly how satan works. If he can't break you and rob you of all your faith and strength, he will have an assistant(s) attempt to rip your faith and strength apart. These two drill sergeants tagged me like a brutish plague for ten weeks! It was both shocking and humbling when I was at the peak of my last week of training and nearly at the end of my boot camp to be called to their office and to be told that I had been selected as an honor to represent my unit at graduation as a part of the American flag folding ceremony.

When I first heard I was to meet with these ruthless drill sergeants in their office, I thought I was in BIG trouble! After all, what could I *expect* from these bullies? An honor, *what* was *that* all about?! Was that satan? Nope! Was that me? Nope. That was God! After their short announcement to me, I said, "Thank you" (as my tears of relief and joy welled up). What do you think the response was? "AS *YOU* WERE! WIPE *THAT SMILE* OFF YOUR *UGLY* FACE!" Umm, as if it was not enough that it was a beaming, hot, humid, ninety-eight-degree day, and rather than the chow from the mess hall sticking to my ribs, it was the sweaty, muddy, starch on my uniform going from stiff to soggy that was now grossly sticking to my ribcage!

Don't dive into satan's faith tests and merciless, pesky discomforts; he's just tempting you to yield into soppy weakness. Soon he will leave you alone because he will find out that you are not easily intimidated by him. And, to his dismay, you are *His* and you rely on *His* strength. *Overcomer*, you are *strong* in Him—*you* are *Overcomer* strong!

SPIRIT MIND BODY

As an *Overcomer*, your mind must think with an attitude of strength and expectancy. Expect your past abuse to become just that—your past abuse. Expect your present *and* future to be abuse-free. God will *always* be there to meet you at your *Overcomer* level of expectancy. If you're expecting something supernaturally good to happen in your life—then that's exactly what is going to happen. If you expect to live a life of inescapable suffering, your own *mindset* and limited expectancy for your life will contribute to the results that you will receive. Whatever your mind thinks, it will expect. Whether you have victim or *Overcomer* expectations, your mind's thinking will set the limits for your life. It's important to note that your expectations as a victim or *Overcomer* fulfills the limits of your faith. Your faith is at work when you surrender your life to God Almighty, and you decide to turn to Him to help you to overcome your abuse. It is your pure act of *mindful* faith and expectancy to become an *Overcomer* that moves God to bring healing to your past.

Matthew 9:29 states: "Then He touched their eyes, saying, 'According to your faith let it be to you.'" What this means is that you shall receive according to your level of faith. The way to start to draw out God's mercy upon you is to put your faith in action. Remaining in the victim's frame of mind (the rut) is not an option for an *Overcomer*. This kind of thinking uses your mind unproductively and only leads to thinking in the wrong direction of darkness. Begin to expect God and the new person within you to make a way and to turn everything around for you in a positive light. That's the right direction for your energies. If you're *not* anticipating that the best is yet to come, and you're spending your time looking back on all of your losses and yet expecting God's supernatural intervention, that approach does not work.

Pay attention to your mind's focus moment-to-moment as you journey in your reality path as an *Overcomer*. Once you reach a level of *Overcomer* status, aim to lose your fear and sustain your mind with faith! Believe that this new life will be lasting because God is going before you to always accompany you and lead the way. *Never* lose heart that once He has done a good thing in your life, you will lose it. Do not revert your mind to victim thinking by ruminating over your setbacks or ominous days. His love, goodness, and promises to you are forever; *you* have to stay in faith forever as well. An *Overcomer's* natural attitude (even though she doesn't feel like it) is one of always coming out better off than before. Your mindful thoughts empower your results.

Our God has the power to allocate divine connections (resources) for you through His supernatural interventions. He is on the lookout for your best interest. Don't listen to others' *voices* of darkness; draw near to His voice of light. God *is* and will *always* be at His throne watching over you—the apple of His eye—for a lifetime. "For thus says the LORD of hosts: 'He sent Me after glory, to the nations which plunder you; for he who touches you touches the apple of His eye'" (Zechariah 2:8). Think about the fact that you are His divine choice and He loves you eternally; to Him, you are valuable! To put it all into perspective, think about what C.S. Lewis and Henri Nouwen once said: It's not about what you think about God; it's about what He thinks of you. God sent His Son to Planet Earth to demonstrate His love for you. You are a divine choice! The Maker of Heaven and Earth sees you and loves you with an everlasting love!

Thinking like and being an *Overcomer* is not a temporal goal; you have to *persist* daily and *persevere* to think about and create an *Overcomer* lifestyle. If you're not expecting to achieve a productive life as an *Overcomer*, then you will lose your enthusiasm and the very reason for getting out of your abusive life. Thank God in advance that you will receive from Him what you request. *Expect* that your request to God will come to pass. What your mind thinks about and expects will be brought about—through God's blessings that will overtake you. Yes, He will bless you abundantly, and while you're thanking Him in advance for upcoming blessings, take a moment to thank Him for your mind and for *all* that He has already done for you. Can't think of anything to thank Him for? Then just thank Him that you're alive. End your prayer that you don't have words for in the following way: "I pray to You in thanksgiving and in His Name, Amen" (even when you've made your prayer requests but everything seems grim). A heart filled with thanksgiving is medicine to your soul. In other words, when your Spirit is filled with gratitude for some details of your life (in spite of all of the pain), your brain chemistry changes and your grateful mind leads to an inner joy in your heart that directs your gestures into a positive attitude (willingness to rest in Him, smile, laugh, and play while you wait for His answers).

God longs for you to rise to a level of an *Overcomer*. God can take you to places that you've never been before, places of tranquility and places that He has placed in your mind and heart through His Spirit. Being an *Overcomer* is pure, heartfelt, peaceful bliss! As an *Overcomer*, God's favor will lead you to overcome *every* obstacle you're faced with—because He desires for you to rise above your circumstances to a level that you've never gone to before—a level of optimum *peace* in your life. God's attention is on defeating your enemy. When you let God into the doorway of your mind, your doorway can now lead you to divine doorways that you *never* knew were there.

These supernatural, mindful doorways have always been available to you; they have your name written on them—it's just a matter of you making up your mind to let God in your doorway first. You will then receive His favor, which has no end, and because you are made in His Image, you can now activate within yourself the mind of Christ through His Spirit. For "Who has known the mind of the LORD that he may instruct Him? But we have the mind of Christ" (1 Corinthians 2:16). You've cried many a tear already. "His favor *is for* life; Weeping may endure for a night, but joy *comes* in the morning" (Psalm 30:5). Go ahead and *ask Him* to walk right into the doorway of your mind and heart. You can trust Him; receive His blessings for a lifetime!

Balancing Your Body
Balancing your body is all about treating your body with respect. A healthy body is one that is not defiled by our self-abuse or the abuse of others. It is a body that is well-nourished with natural and plant-based foods as opposed to processed foods. Plant-based foods have antioxidants and phytochemicals that protect the body from disease. Also, a balanced body is stretched or exercised in between work and other activities; it is a body that develops a high immune system that is resistant to disease.

The victims I have worked with have usually entered my office with a deep need for a lifeline of hope. Their facial expressions and tone reveal their wounded hearts; at times their pain is from both their heart *and* physical body. The despondent look in their eyes is a revelation of their depressed state. Other times, victims were simply infuriated by having lost total control of their Spirit, Mind, and Body. It is certainly humiliating to be treated inhumanely and to lose control of the self. This section is dedicated to those victims that find themselves unable to manage their self and have lost sight of or motivation to take care of their own body. We are going to focus on ways that you can regain control of your body by simply taking good care of it, for the present, *and* investing in good health for the future. I hope you don't skip over this very important part of your journey toward becoming an *Overcomer* and that instead this focus on the body will be a beacon of light for you in balancing your Spirit, Mind, and Body.

SPIRIT MIND BODY

My goal is not to just provide guidelines to improve the functioning of your body—your physical state—but to also equip you with knowledge about *how* the state of your Spirit and Mind affect the state of your Body. Furthermore, the purpose for the information provided is not for it to become a quick-fix but to be practiced daily so that it can become a lifestyle of self-care! At this moment, you may be thinking about how difficult it sounds to focus on taking care of yourself, but the simple truth is that over time, with education, practice, new habit-forming, and discipline, it is possible to rediscover the energy to take care of you. You may not have the motivation to even lift a finger at this time, but the good news is that using energy begets gaining energy. This is a good time to remember the saying: "A journey of a thousand miles begins with one single step." So, let's begin now one step at a time.

People that lead non-abusive lives will always have an edge over others that have suffered the trauma of abuse; they will usually have the remarkable ability to naturally want to and work toward taking care of their body. Like with everything in life, taking care of your body *is* a choice. We will discuss how you can break out of your old way of thinking about your body (postponing the care of it) and *instead* use good judgment in redirecting your thinking toward using your Spirit and Mind to balance and heal your body and mental well-being. One way to break out of not taking care of your body is to begin to create new habits that support the care of you. Research has indicated that it takes twenty-one days to form a new habit. Other experts say that it takes forty days to form a habit and actually even ninety days for that habit to become a natural part of your lifestyle. Whatever the time frame, it is certain that *whatever* you continually think about and practice becomes a habit. So, let's discuss what types of body habits can help a victim as she strides to achieve her *Overcomer* lifestyle—as a natural way of life.

Please understand from the very beginning that you as a victim *or Overcomer* will always encounter distractions (life happens), frustrations, hurdles, and blunders that will lead to mistakes in the habit of taking care of your body. Nevertheless, the foundation of self-care, having been planted, will remain intact, and that base will have already taught you how to incorporate the healthy habit back in when you temporarily fall off-track. The key is that you have to stay on top of becoming aware immediately that you are losing or have lost your bearings (self-discipline) and not allow yourself to back-track and lose permanent ground. How do you regain control of taking care of your body when you're losing ground? Watch out for what your triggers are, which lead you *not* to take care of yourself and gradually go back and incorporate the new behavioral changes (habits) that you have learned.

The behavioral changes that you choose in order to take care of your body are to be committed to for good! They require you to change your mindset about yourself and your body. Body behavioral changes (good body habits) are not to be seen as a part of a season of your life. If you're going to take care of your Spirit, Mind, and Body, the new behavioral changes have to be habitually practiced year-round. You must identify and learn to remove any of the triggers that tempt you to not take care of yourself. What are those triggers that could interfere with your efforts to take care of your body? Take a moment right now to list the triggers that you believe could interrupt you from taking care of your body. The key is to develop a plan as to how you will handle unexpected stressors, interruptions, and other triggers (write down next to each trigger what you will do to counter it). How you handle your triggers is the ultimate acid test that determines your success in taking care of yourself.

One of the behavioral changes that has to be prioritized in order for a victim to take on her role as an *Overcomer* is to make physical exercise a part of her daily living. I know exercise is a bad word to some folks and that time is the number one reason given for not partaking in daily exercise, but a victim just can't afford *not* to make time for this very important step to the balancing of her life. We *all* get the same twenty-four hours a day; it is up to each of us how we divide up our time. Exercise as an abuse trauma intervention is not about looking healthy and fit, although this is one of the fringe benefits of exercise; it is about the benefits of exercising which can directly influence the victim's health and *Overcomer* path. In this sense, it is used as a restorative, curated life approach to treating a traumatized victim. It is an integral part of the life of an *Overcomer* in recovery. Exercise *does not* have to become another overwhelming stressor for the victim; it can actually become a victim and *Overcomer's* friend! This is because if the perception of exercise is one of adding another stressful task to the to-do list, then it will become as such. However, if exercise is perceived as an activity that brings numerous positive results in accomplishing the goal of balancing and obtaining a wholesome well-being, then it's no longer a noxious task to accomplish but a welcome activity that produces healthy feelings and good thoughts.

What are some of the health benefits of exercising that a victim working on becoming an *Overcomer* should consider? Exercise affects your brain. Studies show that when you exercise aerobically there's an increase in the brain's gray matter (the information-processing part of your brain responsible for cognitive and executive function). Executive function is the skill of problem-solving, reasoning, and working memory (working memory stores information for mental tasks). Exercise improves cognitive abilities! Research has shown that exercise can affect thinking and trigger creativity. So, if you're stuck with indecisiveness or searching for a solution to a problem, remember that consistent exercise develops creativity and aids in problem-solving. This means that you can problem-solve to rise above and conquer your abuse by including daily exercise as a strategy to change your habitual thinking as a victim. What we do with our body stays in our soul and in our Mind.

Choosing to stay abused and sedentary is detrimental to your cognitive growth. Your neural pathways will biologically develop parallel to your habits and way of thinking, feeling, and doing. Refraining from getting stuck in your abuse routine can serve to stimulate your stagnant nervous system and develop the growth of new neural pathways, which will form new healthy habits in thinking, feeling, and doing. Exercise has been proven to influence goal-setting and achieving capacities. When a person exercises regularly, this routine accomplishment has a multiple effect in reaching other goals, because a continuation of that activity sets the precedence for developing a desire to try new healthy behaviors. Exercise can inspire the accomplishment of other goals you would otherwise not strive for. When your daily routine includes exercise, your other goals will appear and become more doable and obtainable.

The University of Montreal did some studies which suggest that a moderate twenty-minute workout three days per week during pregnancy boosts a baby's brain development. Since our own brains develop throughout our lifetime, what does that say about exercise and the brain? Exercise increases mental alertness, helps you produce more energy, uplifts your mood, decreases symptoms of anxiety and depression, improves your sleep, balances your appetite, improves metabolism, regulates blood pressure, boosts your immune system (preventing viruses, colds, or flu), aids in digestion, alleviates pain from arthritis or other aches, and helps prevent and protect against major illnesses (heart disease, stroke, diabetes, some cancers). Exercise is a natural benefit as a mood booster and as an antidepressant. This is because exercise alters your nervous system, modifying your levels of hostility and anger (a symptom of hurt feelings). For those that suffer from seasonal affective disorder (SAD), outdoor exercise provides natural sunlight, which can ward off the symptoms of SAD (winter depression).

Exercise can improve the sleep that a victim needs (to restore her energy lost through chronic stress). If you sleep less than six hours daily, your body produces more cortisol (a stress hormone), and that will affect your mood! How is it possible for exercise to improve your mood? Countless research studies have concluded that exercise stimulates endorphins (chemicals actively circulating your body which interact with your brain, providing an overall positive feeling). Exercise sends a message to your brain to release the feel-good endorphins. It's that rush that you feel after an invigorating workout. Endorphins not only impact mood, but they also affect your natural immunity and ability to perceive pain. The other chemical that exercise stimulates is the neurotransmitter norepinephrine, resulting in a total uplift of your mood!

Hopefully, your perspective on exercise is now one that can see exercise as being your friend in helping you reach your goal of becoming a healthy *Overcomer*. As has been discussed throughout this book, how something is *perceived* (positive or negative) makes a tremendous difference on the outcome that follows. The way to have success in exercising to take care of your Spirit, Mind, and Body is to have that powerful *Overcomer* positive attitude! In her book *Prayer Walk*, Janet Holm McHenry talks about the benefits of walking as a form of exercise. She states, "The emotional, spiritual, and physical energy women get from walking powers them through the day." Can a person pray and walk speedily at the same time? Absolutely! Our brain is phenomenal. Whether you choose to pray, focus intensely on your chartered goals, or to envision and daydream about your future enhanced life, all of your positive thoughts calm your *amygdala* (your brain's center for stress/emotions/serenity). When your amygdala's calming alpha waves are increased, the result also directly reduces your levels of cortisol.

How much time should be spent on exercising to reach the coveted, healthy *Overcomer* well-being? Here's some encouraging news for those dreading the time involved in exercise. Most studies have found that thirty minutes of aerobic walking five times per week results in the *same* health benefits (reduction in risks of disease) as running vigorously, provided the walking and running covers the same distance. It's obviously evident that just thirty minutes of daily, brisk walking can achieve the same objective as jogging. It's definitely a matter of your preference as to which form of exercise you prefer.

It's important to remember that it's not about vigorously exercising your body to death. It's *not* about suffering through exercise; it's about benefitting from the exercise. So, have fun while you're out there! Some of my patients have found it more motivating to exercise along with a friend. Brisk or power-walking with a friend (if it's possible with your abusive relationship confines) works well if you both stay on task and do not engage in ongoing conversation which slows down your activity level. If you're able to keep up a fluent conversation and your heart rate is unchanged, then you're not power-walking; you're just taking a constitutional walk. Many find that taking music along as a friend increases their motivation to keep up their exercise pace.

It's noteworthy to add options to your aerobic walking route for the inspirational aspects of experiencing a variety of nature scenery. This will prevent you from getting bored with your routine and losing your enthusiasm for your walks. It's equally important to change routes because your cardio and body muscle needs will change with time, and your body will get used to the routine and no longer gain the aspired benefits. To maintain diversity in your workout, include a variety of paths or trails that have a combination of flat, uphill, and downhill terrain. If brisk walking is not your exercise of choice, there are many other aerobic and anaerobic activities that will accomplish the same health benefits that you are pursuing, such as bike riding (stationary or regular bike), running on a treadmill, using an elliptical machine or stair stepper, dancing, PiYo, Spin, Bungee, or Pilates. The idea is to find an exercise method that you can look forward to and therefore would be willing to do regularly three to five days a week.

Is aerobic activity *all* that is important to partake in in order to improve your mental and physical well-being? No. Strength training is also beneficial for the overall health of your Mind and Body. Finding it difficult to even consider *thinking* about incorporating some strength training into your exercise routine? Perhaps you could look at it from the perspective that it's both for your mental well-being in conjunction with increasing your body's muscle longevity and that it would be a wise investment of your time right about now in your life. The fact that after age twenty-five, adults generally lose around one half to one pound of muscle tissue annually should motivate most of us to take good care of our bodies.

Every ten years after age thirty-five, most adults will naturally lose five to seven pounds of muscle. By the time you reach age sixty, you will have lost approximately twenty-eight pounds of muscle mass that will be replaced by fat. (Our body's usual age progression includes the deterioration of muscle which is then replaced by fat.) In other words, muscle decline is a natural body process, and living an inactive lifestyle not only leaves room for fat replacement, but it also aids in the acceleration of muscle loss. Our body muscle mass has to be used regularly and strengthened daily through deliberate activity if it is to remain intact.

Muscles melting away may not seem alarming when a victim is in the midst of life-and-death problems, but the *truth* is that taking care of your body happens to also be a matter of life and death for any victim or *Overcomer*! Maintaining a healthy body is *not* just about maintaining your muscle mass; it's about keeping your muscle so that your metabolism (which decreases when your body's muscle has been replaced by fat) can work properly. Strengthening muscle tissue involves the regulation of your metabolism, which is responsible for the breakdown of your food consumption and energy levels. For most people, their metabolic rate is responsible for approximately sixty to seventy-five percent of their day's energy expenditure. An *Overcomer* absolutely can't afford not to have her metabolism balanced; her body will function at its best when its metabolic rate is at peak and in balance.

Still wondering *why*, in the middle of resolving the trauma of abuse, a victim or *Overcomer* needs to be on top of her metabolism? Consider the energy levels that our metabolic rate is responsible for; it's the energy that keeps your brain functioning, your lungs breathing, and your heart beating, along with numerous additional cellular processes going on in your body! A metabolism that is regulated by strengthened muscle tissue responds and interacts as a healthy body to the self and the environment. A victim of trauma *and* an *Overcomer* simply can't allow her body to become a place to store fat deposits that do not provide any of the health benefits that she has to have to live a healthy *Overcomer* lifestyle.

This is not about body-building, but again, it is about all of the health benefits that will propel you to carry on as an *Overcomer*. The best way to get the most out of your strength training is to practice *mindful* lifting, similar to *mindful thinking*. Mindful thinking is fully defined in Volume III Part II, but for now, it's simply consciously and intentionally paying attention and becoming fully aware of your experiences in the here-and-now. In strength training, *mindful lifting* involves your full conscious concentration on maintaining proper posture, proper form, correct lifting techniques, and good breathing technique while focusing on keeping your specific muscles engaged in full, gradual movement. The most important part of your strengthening workout is to concentrate on lifting and letting down the weight slowly, focusing on flexing the specific muscle you are aiming to work on with each repetition.

If your circumstances do not allow for weight lifting at home or at the gym, you can still do your aerobic walking and strengthen your upper body through adding wrist weights to your arms. Even three to five-pound dumbbells can be used at home for the strength training of your arms and torso. As with any type of exercise, to reduce the risk of sore muscles and/or injury, always do a five-minute before and after warm-up by doing stretching exercises or using the treadmill or other exercise machine at low intensity. This increases your blood flow to your joints and muscles for your optimum aerobic and/or strengthening workout. Some of my patients have maintained exercise notes in their journal or phone app to assist them by recording their own aerobic activity and strength training workouts; this has served them as an encourager and accountability tool in their body health progress. No time for exercise journaling or phone app activity checkups? Just remember daily that for optimum mental and body health, exercise is a prescription without all of the negative side-effects of medicines; exercise is your go-to medicine of choice!

Shall we proceed to discussing eating habits? We can, but it goes without saying that the focus must also be on balancing nutrition under chronic stress. Without overstating the obvious, you must realize that your nutrition directly impacts the balance of your energy and moods. That is one of the reasons to be mindful of proper nutrition as a victim of abuse. A victim or *Overcomer* with patterns of improper nutrition is like a soldier without a weapon; there's no way that you will be able to fight off any trauma stressors (your enemy) without healthful nutrition. In addition to infilling your Spirit with spiritual food, taking deep breaths and exhaling, calling/texting someone in your support system, and hugging your children—eat healthfully. Eating healthfully improves your blood sugar and hormonal levels—and thus your mood. So take a nutritious meal break and be happy! Who on Earth craves to have an unhappy meal anyway? Studies have found higher levels of depression in people who consume a lot of processed and fast foods compared with those who eat healthy foods. What you eat does impact your stress. For instance, just having walnuts or dark chocolate for a snack can reduce your level of stress hormones!

As a victim of abuse, you're living in (drowning in) chronic stress. Chronic stress lowers a person's metabolic rate, affects sleep and digestion, raises blood pressure, increases breathing and heart rate, and increases *cortisol* levels. Cortisol is a hormone that our body secretes to help us to cope with and provide stamina during periods of stress. When the stress is long-term, such as with the trauma of abuse, the consistent elevation of cortisol levels leads the body to continually release sugar into the bloodstream; this causes insulin levels to rise, signaling the blood sugar to drop. When your blood sugar goes down, your body's response is to increase the production of cortisol. Cortisol causes your body to burn your body muscle as fuel to get you through the stressor. High levels of cortisol not only affect your body muscles, but long-term, trauma-induced stress of any type of abuse deposits large amounts of cortisol that remain in your brain.

This, in turn, can affect various parts of your brain, including damage to the functioning of your hippocampus, which is responsible for your memory system. Cortisol also directly affects the functioning of your neurotransmitters. There are certain foods and beverages that can raise cortisol levels. It is to your advantage to learn the difference between good and bad carbohydrates, as the latter can raise your cortisol levels. Take time to educate yourself through literature and/or the internet on the good nutrients for your body and those foods to avoid. Read labels when purchasing foods. Foods high in bad carbohydrates are high in calories as well *and* lack any source of nutritional value. Look out for various names that are given to sugar: fructose, high fructose corn syrup, or sucrose.

In sum, eating high levels of bad carbohydrates (high glycemic index carbohydrates) such as foods with refined sugars, processed cereals, white flour or rice, and any processed carbohydrates that have been stripped of their beneficial fiber is *not* nutritious for you. The good carbohydrates are full of nutritious fibers, which are absorbed slowly into the body, avoiding the spiking of blood sugar levels which ultimately results in an increased desire for bad carbohydrates (sugar cravings). Good carbohydrates (low glycemic index carbohydrates) include whole grain breads and pasta, beans, vegetables and fruits, and unsweetened juice with pulp—just to name a few. Good carbohydrates provide the vitamins and minerals for body fuel and brain functioning; these are foods that are naturally rich in fiber with the balanced nutrients that are conducive to balancing blood sugar. If you must use sugar, there are natural sweeteners which are made from the sweet extract of the Stevia plant: Stevia, Truvia, and others that contain no calories and are not harmful to your body. Research has found that artificial sweeteners, although they have no calories, *can* contribute to obesity and other serious illnesses.

What role does protein play in balancing your mood and overall physical health? Proteins and amino acids are the units of being for the Body. Proteins and amino acids are responsible for the maintaining and repairing of connective tissue, muscles, skin, hair, nails, and bones. Low levels of protein places you at risk for not being able to maintain these tissues. Furthermore, protein deficiency can affect your blood sugar and hormonal levels, expedite the aging process, deplete your immune system, and make your body more susceptible to disease. Studying which foods contain protein is worth your while! Some proteins to consider are whole grains, nuts, seeds, low-fat dairy products, legumes, eggs, fish, poultry, and lean meats.

What about the fat found in some foods, including proteins? Fat, as is well-known, can affect the overall health of your body. However, it's simple to nip fat in the bud by following a basic fact: It's not about the eating of fatty foods, it's about the type of fat that you consume. There are "good fats" (monounsaturated and polyunsaturated fats), which lower your risk of disease, and "bad fats" (saturated and trans fats), which place you at risk for disease. So, it's a matter of selecting foods that include good fats, such as seeds, nuts, fish, and vegetable oils (olive, canola, sunflower, corn, soy). Our body actually needs certain types of good fats; for instance, Omega-3 fatty acids (which our body is not capable of producing on its own) can be found in fish and other protein foods.

The fats that make the bad list include fatty red meat, whole dairy products, and processed foods that are prepared with trans fats (man-made) from partially hydrogenated oil. Needless to say, if you select foods that have the good fats over the bad fats, and they are consumed in healthy portions, you will not only avoid clogged heart arteries, but you will also feel and experience a healthier body. What's considered a healthy portion? A lot of dieticians advise a visual system using your hand as a measure to guide you. Clenching your fist is about a cup size, which is the amount recommended for a portion of fruit, vegetable, whole grain cereal, pasta, or rice. A lean meat portion is considered to be the size of your palm, and added fats (non-fat dairy products, condiments) are to be the size of the top of your thumb. When you combine good carbohydrates with proteins and good fats in the correct portions, you will experience a calmer mood, a healthy balanced appetite, incredible energy, and both emotional and physical strength.

What about beverages? For excellent mental health and a healthy body, water is your ideal friend in comparison to *all* beverage options. Why? Because water is necessary for producing hormones and neurotransmitters; water delivers nutrients to your brain and transports toxins out of your body! Your brain alone is made up of over eighty percent water; it has to be hydrated with water daily because it does not have the capacity to store water. Water is fuel to your brain; it supplies the brain with energy. In order for your brain to function at optimum levels, it has to have water intake. If you don't drink water every day, you will become dehydrated and may not even realize it until your body begins to exhibit symptoms such as fatigue, foggy thinking, irritability, unprovoked anger, lack of concentration, headache, emotional stress, depression, insomnia, or sleepiness.

Coffee, tea, unsweetened juice with pulp, and non-fat milk, although acceptable beverages to drink in moderation, are not fluids that will keep your brain from dehydration. Notice sodas (regular or diet) were not included in the acceptable beverages list. Most Americans have already been warned that both regular and diet sodas have been associated with increasing the health risks for elevated blood sugar levels, lowering good cholesterol levels, obesity, and heart disease. Your brain can't survive on just intake from these beverages, even if they're considered acceptable fluids; it needs a full reserve of water. It's easy to remember to drink water; you don't have to wait until you're thirsty. Drink water with all of your meals and snacks. One easy way to figure out how much water your own body needs daily is to divide your personal weight in pounds by two. This calculation gives you the amount of water in ounces that your body needs per day to remain hydrated. Keeping your brain hydrated with water will enhance your mental well-being!

Now that we have gone over the importance of balanced nutritious meals for your overall mental and physical health, it's useful to include some factors (triggers) that have to be included in meal planning. Never forget how your triggers, like your environment (social setting), stress levels, and mood, can influence your mind on the choices that you make regarding your and your family's meals. When you detect any of the above-mentioned complex processes interfering with your healthy meal plans, it is time to implement strategies that you have already set in place to debunk stressors or moods that have power over you. Get very acquainted with the cues that can steer you away from your focus on taking care of yourself. This would be a good time to bring to mind some positive affirmations, readjust your environment (or schedule), and do some *mindful thinking* and *mindful eating* instead. Your mindful thinking strategy includes intentionally stocking your pantry, cupboards, refrigerator, and freezer with *only* the foods that will nourish you to health.

Also, mindful thinking recognizes that skipping meals is not an option because it only derails your objective of taking care of your Spirit, Mind, and Body. While you may be able to justify skipping a meal(s), it is not a solution-based strategy to alleviate any unexpected crisis. In fact, it can worsen your circumstances through the health hazards that have been articulated. The worst offender is skipping breakfast as it is the meal that determines your metabolism for the remainder of your day. Whatever you eat or don't eat at breakfast will send a message to your brain about how your metabolism is to break the food down. If at breakfast you eat bad carbohydrates or skip the meal, your brain will signal your metabolism to raise your blood sugar level, reduce your metabolic rate, raise cortisol levels, and anything you eat later will be converted to fat (even if you choose a healthy, balanced meal later). Any time you skip meals, it not only affects your blood pressure and blood sugar levels but your mood as well. An *Overcomer's* goal is an upbeat, positive mood, not a downswing mood. Instead of dealing with runaway thinking (overthinking), biological symptoms, guilt, and other aftermaths of skipping meals, prepare yourself to overcome possible *triggers* that prompt you to skip. If you're unable to consume a meal, then tide yourself over with a nutritious snack.

Keep your handbag, locker, office desk/fridge, or vehicle stocked with healthy snacks that raise your norepinephrine and serotonin levels (see discussion on neurotransmitters that follows). Have snacks prepared and packed in re-sealable plastic bags to take with you wherever you go. Again, healthy snacks include fruits, seeds, nuts, raisins, fat-free Greek yogurt, or low-fat cheese. If you crave more of a meal during snack times, prepare boiled eggs or broiled chicken or turkey in advance; they're packed with tryptophan, which brings on a relaxed state. Tryptophan is an amino acid that produces serotonin, which brings on feelings of contentment and tranquility. Enriched cereal that's high in folic acid is another snack or meal that can serve to regulate mood chemicals in the brain. If your stress is so severe that you can't fathom chewing (let alone digesting any solid food), keep undenatured whey protein powder or protein isolate handy to prepare a smoothie with nonfat milk, fruit, and ice. There are also pre-prepared high protein shakes—read labels carefully for high carbs and unhealthy additives or consult with a pharmacist. It is imperative that you do some positive self-talk or relaxation technique(s) to redirect your focus into a more calmed state so that you will be able to absorb your protein.

Chronic stress affects how protein is absorbed into the body; it impairs your body's ability to digest proteins. Chronic stress levels lead to disease. Maintaining your protein levels will strengthen your immune system. Using *mindful thinking* leads to *mindful eating* naturally. Mindful thinking will provide you with an awareness of the foods, beverages, and portions that you are choosing and consciously consuming daily. Choosing to nourish your body with nutritious meals will benefit both you *and* your children as they learn to habitually take care of their own bodies by watching you. If you're having an especially stressful week, take a sunrise solitude porch or kitchen table coffee/tea break to de-stress yourself. Someone once said that coffee is Jesus' good morning kiss to us! If you're not an early riser, take that break as soon as you are able to be alone. It will restore you back into mindful thinking and eating. A large Harvard University study found that women who drank two cups of coffee daily, compared with those that did not, had a fifteen percent lower risk of depression. Caffeine triggers a release of dopamine which then signals your brain to improve its outlook. So take a coffee break!

A simple sixty-second relaxation technique that can reduce your stress is to take six breaths and exhale. Within one minute your brain will leave the fight, flight, or freeze state and flood your brain with improved mood neurotransmitters. If you're frequently experiencing stress that immobilizes you, try sitting down, place your left hand over your heart, and visualize Jesus holding your right hand, take three slow breaths, and exhale. Initially your heartbeat will be pumping high, but as you exhale after your third breath, you will notice your heart rate has slowed down, and you will be at a more relaxed, peaceful state. For most, it is comforting when they envision their hand is clasped in His. If you feel uncomfortable envisioning holding Christ's Hand, that's okay, you don't have to, although He does promise to hold your right hand: "For I, the LORD your God, will hold your right hand, Saying to you, 'Fear not, I will help you'" (Isaiah 41:13). If you're ever ready to imagine holding His Hand, know that He does not interpret you as silly for imagining clasping His Hand in yours. To clasp Christ's Hand in return is to communicate your trust that He cares about your welfare, and that by faith you can be confident that He will lead you through the wilderness of your abuse, to the doorway of His eternal care for your Spirit, Mind, and Body.

Most victims and *Overcomers* find it useful and gain more success in taking care of themselves by having a friend keep them accountable on their health commitment. Keep in touch on a regular basis via phone, email, private social media page, or in person with someone whom you can count on to provide you with the support and strength that you need to stay on track. Having an accountability buddy will help you to come to grips with whatever your triggers are and help *you* to be accountable to yourself. Your accountability support system can also help to bring things into perspective and enlighten you on the reality of your current circumstances so that you can go back to taking care of yourself. If you don't have a friend that is willing to hold you accountable, remember that through this book, I am *your friend*. Use this book as a go-to and re-read portions that speak to you whenever you want to regain your willpower. Always remember that isolation and a sedentary lifestyle not only breeds depression, but it's also your abuser's wish to isolate you from a support system. Prepare for action!

Let's talk about that moody depression—something that the abuser likes to operate and control. If we *know* this, and we also know that your moods can determine how you feel about you and the care of your body, then it's important to evaluate what kind of moods drive you to not care about taking care of your body. Anger, anxiety, depression, irritation, frustration, physical illness, *and* overwhelming chronic stress can *all* lead you to apathy about yourself. These can all become triggers that tempt you to give up and not take care of yourself.

Menstruation, pregnancy, perimenopause, and menopause can *all* trigger emotional and physical responses. Hormonal imbalances can lead to psychological and physical reactions. Emotional and physiological responses (moods and physiological triggers) *can't* be controlled without balancing the brain and body chemistry. For example, there are three neurotransmitters that can quickly boost or drop your mood. *In order to control mood swings, it's highly important to balance your brain's neurotransmitters.* Some family physicians will not order lab tests for neurotransmitters and will often make a referral for the lab tests to be ordered by a psychiatrist. Ooh, I said a bad word. Psychiatrists are not as bad as they are made out to be; I have worked extensively with and befriended some very fine psychiatrists. Please rest assured that psychiatrists are *not* the stereotyped psychotherapists that people are referred to when they are *crazy*. Psychiatrists are medical doctors that can order tests for neurotransmitter imbalances as well as provide therapy.

The neurotransmitters worthy of evaluating when you're struggling with chronic stress and a mood disorder are *norepinephrine, serotonin,* and *dopamine. The following are the neurotransmitters that you can, with the proper steps, learn to balance:*

Norepinephrine—A deficiency in norepinephrine is closely associated with depression. Low levels of norepinephrine bring on a lack of motivation, increased appetite, cravings for starchy foods, distractibility, difficulty starting or finishing tasks, feeling "blah" or gloomy, lethargic feelings, and ongoing fatigue. Norepinephrine helps a person pay attention to stay alert; it provides the ability to sustain concentration and focus.

Serotonin—Low levels of serotonin are also associated with anxiety and depression. A deficiency in serotonin can lead to insomnia, an inability to relax, obsessive compulsive disorder, irrational behavior patterns, anxiety, panic attacks, irritability, moodiness, premenstrual syndrome, cravings for sweets or starchy foods, and/or eating disorders. Serotonin is known as the "feel happy" or "feel good" neurotransmitter. Generally people with a serotonin deficiency seek activities or relationships that will nurture their need to feel good.

Dopamine—Dopamine is the neurotransmitter that handles anything to do with pleasure. A consistent deficiency in dopamine places the person at risk for becoming addicted to any source of pleasure (work, money, sex, cigarettes, alcohol, drugs, gambling, shopping, TV/media games, food, sleeping, and/or isolation). Chronic stress reduces dopamine. Low levels of dopamine bring on cravings for salty or fatty foods, mood swings, low tolerance for frustration, irritability, forgetfulness, and excessive sleeping. Most people with a dopamine deficiency can become apathetic, procrastinate, and don't have much enthusiasm for anything; they can become moody and depressed and seek pleasure in things to pacify their downcast feelings.

Low levels of *any* of the neurotransmitters in your brain can have a major impact on how your Spirit, Mind, and Body function. Too often victims of abuse trauma are prescribed anti-anxiety or antidepressant drugs to treat the symptoms of a neurotransmitter deficiency which has *not* been diagnosed. This is very counterproductive and ineffective for a victim or *Overcomer* because when the drugs prescribed do not work, their chronic stress increases and may even cause neurotransmitter levels to drop even lower. Testing neurotransmitter levels can get to the root of the neurochemical problem.

There are natural supplements and medications available to balance neurotransmitters. Two neuroscientists, Judy Wurtman, PhD and her spouse, Richard Wurtman, MD at the Massachusetts Institute of Technology, found that there are carbohydrate snacks that can boost serotonin levels in the brain. For instance, eating the correct portion of good carbohydrates can assist in relieving the desire for sugar and bad carbohydrates, ultimately leading the body into producing balanced serotonin levels. Be *mindful*, however, to take into account that when protein is consumed alone (without a good carbohydrate) or in excessive amounts with a carbohydrate, the brain does not produce serotonin. To power-up your brain's serotonin levels and improve your moods, consider one or two snacks daily (approximately three hours post-lunch). Snack on about twenty to thirty grams of whole-grain carbohydrate with less than three grams of fat and less than three grams of protein (low protein portion so it does not reduce serotonin production). It normally takes the average person about thirty minutes after the power snack for the serotonin effect to improve your mood.

Eating nutritious meals, exercising, and taking neurotransmitter supplements combined with mindful thinking can be instrumental in treating a neurotransmitter imbalance. Antianxiety and antidepressant drugs have many side effects that only complicate the symptoms of a neurotransmitter deficiency. If you're experiencing any of the neurotransmitter deficiency symptoms that have been described, it would be to your benefit to be tested to verify if you have a deficiency. If you want to be tested (but prefer not to be tested through a local physician and lab), you can go on the internet and order a non-invasive urine lab test to check your neurotransmitter levels. Go to www.neurorelief.com. After you receive your test results, talk to your physician about the natural treatment options he would recommend.

As has been pointed out, a neurotransmitter deficiency *does* include symptoms of depression. Some symptoms of depression are indeed responses to present/past trauma, physical illness, and/or grief. For some individuals, depression can remain dormant for days, months, or years as the individual goes about their daily life. Then one day, the individual becomes aware of their underlying depression as it surfaces to their consciousness. There are unlimited psychological and physiological factors that contribute to depression (e.g. chronic stress, unresolved trauma, hormonal imbalances, medications, sleep or eating disorders, head injury, brain chemical imbalance and more). Other individuals have a genetic clinical depression. However, even if an individual has a family genetic predisposition for depression, it *does not* mean that the other psychological, physical, and/or environmental factors that contribute to the depression cannot be intervened. Individuals suffering from the trauma of abuse definitely have more than genetic symptoms of depression to treat. Physician, author, speaker, and health and fitness scientist, Pamela Peeke, has been known to say, "Genetics may load the gun, but environment pulls the trigger."

I like the statement that one of the animated characters, Khalil, in *Jonah: A Veggie Tales Movie*, makes about family disposition. When Khalil appears on the screen, he has huge headphones through which he consistently listens to positive affirmations. One of his affirmations is: "You do not run from your problems but confront them face-to-face." Khalil introduces himself as: "I'm Khalil. I'm a caterpillar. My mother was a caterpillar, my father was a worm, but I'm okay with that now." Throughout the movie, Khalil claims *all* of the positive attributes declared by anyone and then repeatedly states: "It runs *very deep* in my family." Is Khalil in denial of his family of origin or a proficient liar? Neither—the message to the audience is that when it comes to family genetic predisposition, it's all about the *attitude* that you take.You can choose a healthy outcome!

Environment can definitely be superimposed, but if we *know* the environment is unhealthy for us, then we *can* work to remove ourselves from that environment. The environment we surround ourselves with can determine what happens to us. What we listen to can impact our decision-making and attitude.

Even though all of the scenes in the movie involving Khalil are done humorously in tongue-and-cheek, the movie does its job in delivering a powerful message to the viewer as Khalil goes around with his huge headphones, listening to ultra-optimistic affirmations and displaying his *Overcomer* attitude. A victim *can override* her genetic predisposition to trauma and depression by *choosing* an *Overcomer lifestyle* and surrounding herself with healthy choices that optimize the health of her Spirit, Mind, and Body. The bottom line for *most* victims of trauma is that mindful thinking and balancing the neurotransmitters, combined with individual and/or group therapy, bring optimum relief from the triggers of clinical depression.

Let's have a word about vitamins and hormonal supplements. There are (and there will always be) some questionable vitamin supplements and hormone replacement therapies out on the market, but there are also arrays of safe and highly effective supplementary vitamins *and* hormones. Most of the research indicates that complete multimineral vitamins with fruits, vegetables, and antioxidants that are formulated for women of specific age groups work well to support energy and the immune system. Another supplement that has been researched and found to optimize well-being is the Omega-3 fatty acids in foods or fish oil capsules. Omega-3 has not only been recommended to prevent various illnesses, but it has also been found to assist those that experience depression. Let us now discuss hormonal balances.

Why do we want to discuss hormones in the middle of dealing with victim abuse trauma? Primarily because hormones evolve from your brain—the very important center of your well-being. For our brain to function adequately, it must have balanced hormonal levels. Women of all ages can experience hormonal deficiencies, *especially* those undergoing chronic stress. A woman's functioning and well-being can be influenced by hormonal imbalances. For example, the female hormone *estrogen* helps to balance the neurotransmitters in the brain, aids in regulating blood sugar levels, sleep, metabolic rate, maintains muscle mass, memory, appetite, mood, weight, prevents osteoporosis, and regulates premenstrual, menstrual, and menopausal symptoms.

Progesterone is another female hormone equally desirable at optimal level. If progesterone levels are down, the person is then susceptible to premenstrual syndrome, depression, decreased libido, mood swings, hair loss, insomnia, anxiety, menopausal symptoms, infertility, and other medical complications. Other crucial hormones to consider evaluating and getting laboratory tests done on are the thyroid hormones. A lot of family physicians overlook the thyroid and instead diagnose the patient with chronic fatigue or depression. When evaluating and getting tested for your hormones, keep in mind the fact that even if you get the proper treatment to balance hormonal deficiencies in estrogen and progesterone, your symptoms may not be relieved due to neglecting to evaluate for a thyroid disorder.

All of these hormones work together to deliver your brain output. In order to evaluate hormonal balances, it is imperative that you find a board certified physician that is well-versed and trained in hormone replacement. Some gynecologists will not prescribe hormone replacement. Doing the physician research will ascertain you of proper testing and that if a deficiency is found, the physician will not attempt to treat you with hormones which have been found to have adverse side effects and add health risks to your body. Hormones that are extracted from plants are healthier. Just like it is healthier not to eat processed foods and to ingest plant-based foods instead, it is also healthier to choose plant-based hormones! It's the natural process from where the hormones are derived that safeguards so that the molecular structure of the hormones is compatible (identical) to the natural human hormones that are produced in the body (in the ovaries, adrenal gland, and hypothalamus).

The first step (once you find a qualified physician) is to be tested for your levels of estrogen, progesterone, and thyroid. If you're unable to locate a physician in your area that offers hormone replacement, you may want to get a referral from the Women In Balance website www.womeninbalance.org or www.worldhealth.net.

It is your lab report that will indicate *if* and *where* there's a hormonal deficiency that needs to be balanced. You, your physician, and your pharmacist can work together to restore hormonal balance to your system. Natural supplements, vitamins, and balanced hormones that are armed with proper exercise, nutritious eating, mindful thinking, and spiritual growth can assist you in realizing that yes, you *can* take good care of yourself! You *can* break free from your maladaptive patterns. You, too, can have a healthy body for life!

Let's get back to our discussion about taking care of your body as a *choice*. The only exception that is *valid* in choosing to *not* take care of your body is when your abuser threatens your safety if you exercise, so you choose to protect you and your children by adhering to his request. This would be an opportunity to process in your mind (and seek assistance from a resource) if you're willing to live with such restraints for the rest of your life. Yes, the abuser has a way of turning your life into a roller-coaster of moods, and after a while, it becomes foggy as to why you should even bother taking care of yourself. While working with victims, I have encountered many a victim stuck in that type of self-defeating mindset, which sabotages whatever glimpse of hope she had of restoring her well-being. There is a way out of this dark victim abyss.

The truth is that your most powerful obstacle is *not* just your abuser; it is also your *mindset*. And guess what? It is satan's mindset as well because your body is the temple of the Holy Spirit, and *he* couldn't care less if the abuser or you choose to destroy it. Take a close look at the following excuses for not taking care of your body: "I don't have the energy" (learn how to gain energy), "I don't have time" (make time), "I can't do it alone" (find a buddy), "my friends and family don't care" (find a resource that does). Do you see the hazardous potential for a downward spiral in your goal to take care of yourself with that mindset? That kind of mindset is self-destructive, and it further entraps the victim into not taking care of herself and propels the blaming of others for her circumstances, ultimately seeing herself as a dismal failure (fulfilling the abuser's prophesy). This can culminate to a point of resignation from taking care of the self. Victims and *Overcomers* who take care of their bodies simply have taken responsibility for themselves. Taking care of the self is a choice which empowers a person to develop lifelong healthy habits.

The time to start to take care of you is *now*. There will never come a time when all the lights will be green—that's unrealistic thinking. Please understand that the very reason that you selected this book to read is reason enough to believe that *you are ready* to make choices and changes. Taking care of your body will provide you with the gift of health, which can bring self-confidence, hope, and *peace* during a traumatic time in your life. Your life as a victim is up-in-the-air; taking care of you can give you assurance of a balanced lifestyle as an *Overcomer*. If taking care of you becomes a choice in your heart, then you will have the outcome of a healthy *Overcomer* lifestyle. But, if your mindset is strictly on your negative abusive relationship and you ignore your body and health, then whatever you focus on the *most* is what you and your life will become.

This leads us to a discussion on visualization and affirmations. When you venture into developing a new habit, you can think your mind into positive visions of yourself and actively encourage your heart to ascertain your successful level of performance by giving yourself self-talk (affirmations). This self-talk must be in the second-person pronoun so that it releases a powerful, motivational pep talk to your brain. For example: "You've got this!" "You can finish this!" "You can conquer this!" There's a behavioral change advantage when one's attitude is prepared in advance of the task with a positive, achievement-minded approach. Personalizing your self-talk by adding your name to the "you" self-talks strengthens prospective behavioral-intended performance. For example, think, "Jane Doe, you can do this!" Giving yourself "you" self-talk is simply giving yourself good advice that you would preferably want to follow as opposed to having a blank slate or listening to your negative self-talk advice. Your positive thoughts and self-talk are nutritiously nourishing to your Mind just like food is to the Body.

The Psalmist knew thousands of years ago about the importance and results of an affirmation. In Psalm 119:11a, he states, "Your word I have hidden in my heart." Hiding God's Word in his heart meant he was memorizing and meditating on Scripture to guide his thoughts and behavior. You too can use power verses as affirmations that inspire, encourage, comfort, and motivate you into action. Select the verse and write it in your phone notes, PC screen page, Post-It note in your car, or wherever you will see it frequently. For example: "I will praise You, for I am fearfully *and* wonderfully made; Marvelous are Your works, And *that* my soul knows very well" (Psalm 139:14). Your body is wonderfully made! "If you abide in Me, and My words abide in you, you will ask what you desire, and it shall be done for you" (John 15:7). Do you believe that? While you're alone, reflect upon a verse that you have selected and written down to hide in your heart. Allow the verse to gently work in your heart. The key is to read each word in the verse slowly, while feeding your soul and transforming your being. The benefits of reading at a slower pace is that you begin to learn the verses by heart and you are able to use the verses as encouraging affirmations as needed.

SPIRIT MIND BODY

Whatever your mindset consistently confesses and visualizes—you will be. Frequently visualize yourself as having a healthy Spirit, Mind, and Body, always remembering "Whose" you are and "Whom" you serve! Imagine yourself as an *Overcomer*, and speak only positive affirmations to yourself. This will help you reach your goal of taking care of you. Do not make a habit of speaking weak "*I*" self-talk statements such as, "I want to," "Sometime I will," or "I'm planning on..." Otherwise, you will remain in the lack of, wanting sometime, planning stages for a lifetime! Instead, say aloud: "You are____," "You have____," "You can__," or "You will___." As you make these affirmations about the care of your body throughout your day and as you begin to follow through, you will start building a habit that you will naturally become attracted to, and you will, in turn, develop healthy behavioral patterns.

Will you be caught off-guard every now and then with your feelings in the midst of working to get out of an abusive lifestyle? Yes. That is precisely why it is crucial if you are to take care of yourself that you begin to identify how you are feeling daily. The reason for this is because, as was stated earlier, our feelings can impact our thoughts and actions. If you ignore your feelings, you will not be able to evaluate the status of your thoughts, and you will have no control over your actions (your body). For example, when you're feeling poorly, it is an indicator of having negative thoughts. Generally, toxic thoughts bring on negative feelings. In the same way, if you're feeling good, you're usually thinking positive thoughts. Taking time out daily to ask yourself how you're feeling increases your awareness of whether you're feeling good or not. This daily evaluation searches your mind as to whether you're thinking positive or negative thoughts. It's not possible to have toxic thoughts throughout the day and experience happy feelings at the end of the day. In other words, you can't have a negative mindset and experience good feelings at the same time. The advantage of evaluating your thoughts throughout the day gives you the opportunity to use the tool of deliberately changing your mindset to optimistic thoughts in order to change your feelings (mood) to a more positive outlook; therefore, this empowers you to change your actions (what your body ultimately does).

There are no wonder-working physical or therapeutic approaches to balancing your Spirit, Mind, and Body; those are shortsighted approaches. With *mindful, long-term thinking,* there is hope for a victim in balancing her Spirit, Mind, and Body while she *works* on becoming an *Overcomer*. A balanced Spirit, Mind, and Body are essential in strengthening your abilities successfully; it also invites the art of tranquil recreation into your inner world. Seeking that necessary mental strength feeds your positive self-image, motivates you, and gears you up to persevere and to follow through as an accomplished *Overcomer*. A lifestyle of regular inspirational and spiritual living, exercise, balancing hormones/neurotransmitters, eating healthier nutritious snacks/meals, accountability, and support is the answer!

As a rookie *Overcomer*, it is vital that you practice a balanced wellness plan which includes being nurturing and kind to yourself while experiencing the transition from your trauma into overcoming your abuse. It is as if you have gone through surgery, and the cancer of abuse has been removed. When someone has surgery, they are cared and provided for through nutrition, nurturing, and especially planned activities that improve their well-being. You must not over-function nor deny that a major life change has taken place and carry on with everyone else's needs or expectations of you and doing business as usual. You are a recovering victim transitioning as an *Overcomer*, and you deserve to be understood just like the person that has had surgery (attended to with respect and soothing compassion).

So, treat yourself with loving wellness-care. Take time out to enjoy doing what you like to do, especially when you're feeling stressed. Have a trusted friend watch the children while you have some alone time or entertainment. Your healing process is more important than meeting others' demands of your person (which then puts you at risk for neglecting your well-being). Solitude as a part of self-care can be healing. Make a final decision to only allow healthy habits into your life.

Healthy habits neurologically grow your Mind. Decide to live a curated life. Living a curated life means being choosy as to what or whom you will permit to influence, mold, and develop your Mind, environment, health, relationships, and identity. It is about never surrendering your worth, and it is always about maintaining its well-being. You do not live in the past except to learn from the past; instead, you curate your present life as needed and live in it *peacefully* with a strong *faith* and a *hope* for your future.

If you have now reached a point of being determined to take care of your Spirit, Mind, and Body, and it's the strongest or most resolute step that you've *ever* known before, then I'm smiling and glad for you! I bet that you sense *some* joy in having made that decision. I'm happy that you have chosen to begin self-care with some resolve compared to other attempts that you may have already made.

However, it's important for you to understand that joy and determination are emotions. Emotions and willpower are *not* sufficient in and of themselves to meet your goal because these are human feelings that can be intruded upon and even evaporate over time. How can you use this new resolve and these feelings of joy and momentum as a powerful motivational force during those times that your abuser or others wreak havoc in your life? You add a *covenant* to those feelings!

When you make a *covenant* to yourself to take care of your Spirit, Mind, and Body, it's like having a pledge, promise, and commitment to yourself; it's a *contract* with yourself. A covenant goes beyond a goal; it allows you to forgive yourself when you back-track. You're able to reprogram yourself to the commitment outlook; it allows you to visualize this commitment as long-term, and therefore you return to your undertaking when and if you lose your determination.

Making a covenant to yourself will reassure you of not ending up in the same place you have been before as a victim while operating from a victim mindset. The difference with having a covenant is that you're no longer just saying to yourself that you're going to take care of your Spirit, Mind, and Body, but you're *actually* going to sign your *Covenant* as your commitment to take care of yourself. Most victims and *Overcomers* have their designated support person sign as a witness who will hold them accountable. *Overcomers* usually place their Covenant in a designated strategic area which they can see daily.

The Covenant puts your goal in a positive framework as opposed to viewing it as another laborious task list. It's drafted and drawn to personally benefit you; it targets and focuses on the achievement of your *Overcomer* goal. Can an *Overcomer* balance her Spirit, Mind, and Body *without* making any adjustments and/or changes to her health habits and just take a risk on the outcome? No, that's not for you; taking risks on destructive outcomes is no longer in your thinking patterns. If you want to balance your Spirit, Mind, and Body, you have to put the brakes on living your life with mindless thinking.

Although your Spirit, Mind, and Body covenant is between you and God and may appear like an ordinary piece of paper, it has been known to be a powerfully symbolic written document that leads a person to maintain their commitment. The covenant is set in place as a vision and backup commitment for when your feelings fluctuate and turn against your goal. The covenant also serves as a tool and reminder that you have the power to choose your thoughts; you can write or verbalize them and substitute positive thoughts for toxic ones. The covenant is like your declaration of independence to run and balance your own Spirit, Mind, and Body. The covenant represents your choice to live a curated life. Are you ready to sign your *Overcomer Spirit, Mind, and Body Covenant*?

Spirit Mind & Body Covenant

I, _____, hereby sign this covenant as my pledge to take care of my Spirit, Mind, and Body from this day forward.

- ✓ I commit to secure a friend or other resource to hold me accountable.
- ✓ I commit to an inspirational, quiet, spiritual time of no less than fifteen minutes daily.
- ✓ I commit to evaluate my thoughts daily and substitute realistic, positive thoughts for toxic thoughts.
- ✓ I commit to remove all non-nutritious foods from my refrigerator, freezer, and pantry.
- ✓ I commit to respecting, being kind to, and nurturing myself daily.
- ✓ I commit to brisk walking or another form of exercise for at least thirty minutes three to five days a week.
- ✓ I commit to maintaining journal progress notes or a fitness app to record and balance my nutrition, exercise, and activities.
- ✓ I commit to visualizing myself daily as a healthy *Overcomer* with a balanced Spirit, Mind, and Body.
- ✓ I commit to positive self-talk through second person pronoun affirmations about taking care of my Spirit, Mind, Body, and speaking affirmations aloud.

I am aware and completely understand that my failure to comply with this Covenant sabotages my *Overcomer* goal to take care of myself. I agree to adhere to *all* of the above commitments that I have made in order to reach my goal of balancing my Spirit, Mind, and Body.

Your signature: _____ Date: _____

Supportive witness signature: _____ Date: _____

> "Then the LORD answered me and said: 'Write the vision and make *it* plain on tablets, that he may run who reads it.'"
> **Habakkuk 2:2**

CASSANDRE'S STORY

OTIS ENTERED MY LIFE during my teen years. Both of us grew up in the ghettos of New York; most people just call it *Harlem*. We met in high school during my junior year and his senior year. I went to our high school basketball game (at which he was playing) with a few of my girlfriends. After the game, I saw him at the local pizza hangout. Otis came over to me and introduced himself; he commented on how beautiful I was and that he would love to take me out sometime. I smiled and gave him my phone number—he didn't hesitate to call. Once on the phone that evening, I let him know that before he could take me out on a date, he would have to meet my mama. I told him that I had been allowed to date since age sixteen but that one of the conditions was getting my mama's approval and that I was not allowed to go out on school nights.

My parents migrated to New York City from Haiti. When my dad became terminally ill, my mama had to move out of our nice neighborhood. My four siblings and I were distraught to leave our friends and transfer to not-so-nice schools, but we got used to it. We lost our dad when we were all in elementary school.

Otis' parents were raised in Detroit, Michigan, and according to what he said, they were actually upgrading when they moved to Harlem. Otis has two siblings; he had three, but one of them died in a drive-by shooting. I brought Otis home to meet Mama after one of our basketball games. She was polite to him and said, "It's fine if you all get together as a group to go out, but as far as just the two of you, I'm gonna have to get to know you better, boy!" After Otis left, Mama said that she didn't like the way Otis had flared up in his temper when she had seen him before (with his peers and coaches). Mama had gone to the games when I was cheerleading; that's how she remembered Otis. I argued with Mama that night and told her it wasn't fair for her to judge my friends. I ignored Mama's preference that I only see Otis with groups of friends; I started seeing him behind her back any time I could. I would leave the house to go out with friends, but instead I would meet him, and we would hang out. Everyone else but Mama came to know us as a couple. I had practically abandoned my friends, even my best friend.

Otis respected me, except once in a while when he got impatient and wanted to go all the way; I broke up with him a couple of times because of that. Otis kept saying it was okay to be close because he wanted to marry me. I told him that if he was that serious about me, we had to go see Mama again. Otis was getting ready to graduate with no plans to go to college—he said he didn't know what he wanted to do with his life. I still had one more year to graduate, but I knew what *I* wanted to do! More than anything, I loved fashion! I wanted to study fashion and design. I told Otis that if he was going to be talking marriage, he better have a job before even thinking about going to see Mama. Otis got a job working at some kind of mail box store part-time, with an agreement to work full-time after graduation. Call me head-over-heels in-love or just on cloud nine because I couldn't understand why my friends, teachers, and just about *anyone* would say that we were much too young to marry! I kept reminding them that we would graduate first, that we were in love, and that we were both very mature for our ages. Otis and I were both in denial, assuming that Mama would hear us out. Otis said he couldn't get me an engagement ring but that he would, eventually, when he got some money. I said, "That's okay."

I will never forget the hurt look on my mama's face when we called a meeting with her; she knew now (without me saying anything) that I had defied her. She treated Otis kindly while she sat down with us at the kitchen table. She silently passed him a piece of her homemade apple pie. Mama's eyes got very sad and glazed when Otis asked for my hand in marriage. She said, "You kids do whatever you want to do because you're going to do it anyway, but I think you both should *wait* to get to know each other better. Marriage is a sacred thing and a *huge* responsibility, and I just don't think either of you are ready for it. No, you don't have my blessing." We kept justifying that we were going to wait until I graduated, that Otis had a job, that I would get a job, and that I would go to technical school. Mama asked me if I had met Otis' family; I said, "no, ma'am." This didn't go over well with Mama—she then said, "I don't have anything further to say; sounds like you've made up your minds to marry without even knowing what you're getting into." Mama got up from the table and washed our dessert dishes.

The next time the subject was brought up was after my graduation, when I told Mama we were going over to get our marriage license. My relationship with my mama had never been the same since I took up with Otis. Mama and my sisters had always had good mother-daughter relationships, but I had messed up mine by ignoring her advice. By now, I had barely met Otis' parents. Otis took me to meet them one night after he got off work. We waited a while for his mother to get home. We almost left without meeting his father because his mother didn't know where he was or what time he would be home. I smelled liquor in his father's breath when he shook my hand. Otis told them that we wanted to get married by the end of summer. Both of them responded like a chorus and said, "Is that right?" Nothing more was said. Otis took me home; we sat outside in his car making wedding plans.

We had to go through some kind of Catholic pre-marriage sessions with a priest because I was Catholic. I don't even have a clue what those were all about! It was just mumbo-jumbo to me. Otis had to become Catholic to marry me or they wouldn't marry us. Otis agreed to become Catholic because he didn't have a religion anyway. Our wedding was small with only some friends and family; we had a punch and cake reception in my home. I wore my mama's vintage wedding dress which I had claimed since childhood; she was gracious to allow me to wear it after I had disappointed her with Otis. It seemed like everything for the wedding and reception was something borrowed. But we were so very happy and that's all that mattered to us. We rented a one-room kitchenette apartment. We did everything in that one room: ate, slept, bathed, and watched a TV with three channels (we bought it at the Goodwill).

I found a sales job at a boutique; I was so excited! Otis was very frustrated because I had to travel on the subway to the upscale parts of New York (it was over an hour commute). Whenever I got home, he would be so upset because it was dark out; he said I had no business out on the streets late at night especially when my man was at home hungry! Every day we were either fighting about my job, or, we would argue because I was saving up to go to a fashion and design school; he thought that I should not give him just *part* of my check, but my *entire* paycheck because he paid the bills. Otis wouldn't yell at me all of the time. Mostly he would, in a quiet tone—lower than his usual voice—let me know that he was angry at me and would say, "You better straighten-up and hear me out, girl!" Other days, he would be sitting in the apartment with the lights out and would greet me with, "It's about time you got home." I would turn the lamp on, and he would say, "Did I say you could turn the light on?" I would say, "Otis, I'm going to trip in the dark. Besides, I have to fix dinner; I need the light." Otis would make me apologize for being home from work after dark; he would make me *plead* to have the lights on in the apartment.

This attitude and arguing went on for over a year; he would sit and sulk or pout because I wouldn't change jobs. Most days, he wouldn't talk to me. The only time he didn't give me the silent treatment was when he wanted to go to bed with me; he would apologize for being moody and come home with flowers or chocolates. This was so hurtful to me, instead of soothing, because he would argue or become sarcastic with me the night before and then expected me to be smooching with him the very next night. I was making good money, and we needed both of our incomes, but after a couple of years of nonstop arguing about my job, I settled for a dime store job in our neighborhood. It was depressing because I was making less money, and I couldn't save up for school. I just didn't want to argue anymore—big mistake! The arguing didn't stop; instead, it changed into arguing about something else.

By then, Otis had gotten into a pattern of melancholic quietness; he wouldn't talk to me. Whenever I would inquire if everything was okay, he would say, "Leave me alone." I told him that I loved him, cared about him, and that was the only reason I was asking him if he was okay. Otis then started being the one to come home after dark—only it wasn't because of work. If I asked where he had been, he would say, "None of your business, woman. You stay out of my business!" Many a night I would fix dinner for us, and he wouldn't show up until after midnight. I knew he wasn't drinking because he didn't drink. Otis had made that commitment while growing up; his father had apparently been an alcoholic. Otis said he didn't want to be like him.

One day while I was doing laundry, I smelled fragrance on Otis' shirt. I asked him about it; he said that he and a buddy had gone to play pool and a couple of ugly gals had joined them to play. Otis kept saying, "Oh, but they were *real ugly* mothers!" Otis said, "I guess the fat chick kept hanging on me and had on too much smelly stuff." I forgave Otis for his shirt smelling like a woman. One morning, Otis forgot his cellphone at home. It rang, and I picked it up, thinking it may be him looking for his lost phone. Instead, a woman on the phone asked for Otis. I said, "Otis is at work; can I help you?" I told her that I was his wife, and she said, "Otis said he wasn't married," and then she hung up. After that, I looked through Otis' phone directory, and he had oodles of women's names and contact numbers! I was afraid that Otis would flip his lid if he knew that I had searched through his phone. I just set his phone back down where he had left it. That night, Otis walked in angrier than I had ever known him. Otis said that I had no business talking to anyone about him and that he was stopping *my* cellphone service because he couldn't trust me with *my* cellphone anymore. Otis disconnected my cellphone the next day—the only source of connection that I had with my mama and sisters. I cried myself to sleep that night; I hardly slept a wink. I wasn't allowed to visit my mama and sisters as it was, unless Otis was with me, because he said it was too dangerous for me riding the subways or walking by myself in their neighborhood. I usually argued back on this one because he knew I had walked and ridden the subways to my neighborhood all of my life, and *nothing* had happened to me.

I still had a burning desire to go to fashion design school, but every time I brought it up to Otis, he would blow me away. Once he said, "Why can't you be happy with just *me* baby; aren't I enough for you?" I wanted to tell him how unhappy I was with my job, but I had already said that. I wanted to tell him how I missed having friends, but I had already spoken to him about that. I wanted to tell him how *hurt* I was that I couldn't go visit my family on my own anymore, but I had already told him that. At that point, I decided to ask him if he would want me to have a job that could pay more, but it could be a freelance job that I could set my own hours. Otis said, *"Now* you're talking." I told Otis that while I was working at the boutique, a lady had given me a business card for a modeling agency, and she had told me to give her a call. Otis said it would be okay to check it out, especially if it meant that we could get some money to get out of the rat hole that we were living in.

Everything went well at the agency. I let them know that I couldn't work evening gigs. It was then that Otis allowed me to have a phone again because I would need it for work! Even Otis got a better job with a parcel service. Otis was surprisingly ecstatic when I began to bring home bigger and bigger paychecks. We moved into a one-bedroom apartment in a nice neighborhood closer to my agency, so I could walk over. Otis didn't think I had any business driving; he said he had to have a driver's license for work but that I didn't need a car. Other than Otis arguing with me—because I said that I still would like to have driving lessons—all was well with us. It wasn't long, though, before I was coming home from work and Otis was nowhere to be found! Otis wouldn't say where he had been when he wasn't scheduled to work. It was always bewildering to me how he could be intimate with me all the time, and he still went out on me. I knew he was cheating on me again. Otis was always on the defensive whenever I inquired about his whereabouts. I had also found some pornographic magazines, and he got super angry when I told him I didn't want those in our home. Otis refused to get rid of them; he said he couldn't throw out magazines that weren't his. I once walked in on him while he was in the act with one of those magazines. I was so ashamed of him! I felt personally rejected because all I had ever done was to serve him as his wife; I didn't know what I could do to satisfy him. I wondered why he had to have porn magazines and other women in addition to a wife. Once in a while, he wouldn't come home, and he would tell me to shut up if I asked, "Where have you been, baby?"

One day, I had had the most exciting day in a long time. I had opened up a secret savings account from some checks that I had not given to Otis, and I had noticed that I had enough money in there to register for the fashion design school. I thought *maybe* if Otis was having a good day and was not down in the dumps or arguing about something, I could talk to him about going to school. I was feeling pretty good until I heard laughter coming from our apartment; I walked in on Otis and some random chick that was half naked. I ran out of our building and just walked and walked for blocks, hot tears rolling down my cheeks. I didn't know where I was going, but I just kept walking. I must have walked for over an hour. I couldn't believe what I had seen; the pain of the betrayal of his love was so unbearable. I felt betrayed, humiliated, and unworthy of his love. I can't even begin to describe that deep hurt in my heart. I felt my heart actually physically *aching*.

While walking, all of a sudden, I panicked! I began to worry about how late it was getting and that I needed to walk back before it got dark. Otis was home and said, "Hey baby, I can explain what you saw. I *don't even know* that gal, and she doesn't mean a thing to me; you're more important to me—*you know that*." I told Otis that I had had enough and that he needed to leave, or *I* would have to leave. Otis said, "Then I guess you're leaving." I packed up my things and as I was walking out, he said, "Don't bother using our credit cards because I already closed them while you were packing." I stayed at a hotel that night. When I went to the bank in the morning, Otis had closed our joint checking account. If it wasn't for the cash I had in my wallet and for the savings account that I had secured, I would not have had any money. A friend that I had met at the modeling agency talked to her photographer boyfriend (that she was living with), and they allowed me to stay in their spare bedroom until I could get my head together.

That week, an agent visited our agency who was scouting for models to take overseas for runway and photography modeling. Out of hundreds that auditioned, I was one of the few selected. I was excited, yet my heart was still so broken over Otis. Otis kept calling my agency leaving messages for me to call him because I wasn't returning his calls. I finally called him back just before I left for overseas. Otis pleaded for me to reconsider going overseas and said, "I'll be good, baby, I promise." I told him that I had already signed a contract and that I had to go to do some catalog and runway bookings. My New York agency made the mistake of giving him the phone number to my overseas agency; he manipulated it out of them. Otis told them that he was my husband and that he had some urgent information to give me about my family. Otis called my agency overseas within the first couple of weeks that I was there; he left a message for me to call and said that he was having an emergency.

When I called him back, he had no emergency—just tears, promises of no cheating, and begging for my forgiveness and to return home. I told him I thought that *if* we got back together, we should go to some marriage counseling and *then* decide if we should stay together. I continued to work, even went out to dinners and nightclubbing with some agency friends. But I was still in love with Otis, and I wanted our marriage to work. I called Otis, and we made up over the phone. I was only overseas for six months out of my one-year contract (which they wanted to extend since I was getting so many gigs). The agency was not pleased with my decision to end the contract prematurely; they made me pay back all of the money (from my earnings) that they had invested in my travel and lodging. I came home with some money and was determined to get back to work at my New York agency. I was *devastated* to find out that my New York agency did not want me back because I backed out on my overseas contract. Any agency that I turned to didn't take me once they found out that I broke an agency contract.

The only good news was that Otis and I were back together, just like when we were dating: two peas in a pod. A month went by, and Otis was making excuses as to why we couldn't make it to a marriage counselor, saying, "We're getting along, so why should we have to go?" I told Otis I still thought it would be good to talk about how we could build a strong marriage in spite of the past affairs. Otis, although not yelling, softly got in my face and said, "Why can't you just let go of the past and let the dog die!" I told him that I had forgiven him, or I wouldn't have come back, but that one of the conditions that we had agreed on for my return was that we would go to marriage counseling. Otis said, "Well, I guess you got fooled then. I ain't going to *any* counseling because there's nothing wrong with me; it's *your* problem, deal with it!" My heart was broken *again* because I had to admit to myself that he had lied just as he had done so many previous times, just to get his way! I began to believe for the first time that maybe Otis didn't care about me or love me in the way that he said he did (not in the way that I loved him). I *adored* him. Perhaps he was lying about his love for me as well. After I couldn't get back into any modeling agencies, Otis had said that I didn't need to find a job if I didn't want to because he was making enough money to provide for us through the parcel service. I still wanted to get a job and save money because my heart's desire was to get into fashion design. It was nearing the holidays, so I began to job hunt.

CASSANDRE'S STORY

I got a job at a retail store the first day I went out looking—yay! Otis was furious. I was able to calm him down (never mentioning fashion design school) by explaining that it was temporary and that it would help to have the extra money for Christmas expenses. This job helped to distract me from the loss of my modeling work and Otis' refusal to go to counseling with me. However, I still had to deal with Otis' melancholy mood that he would get into every year at Christmas time. I had never had a happy, *fun* Christmas since I left home and married Otis. Otis said that he couldn't help it that he hated Christmas because his dad left them one Christmas when he was little and didn't return for several years. Otis couldn't bear the sound of Christmas music, so we never played it. I understood Otis' past hurts with his dad. But what I couldn't relate to was why we as a couple had to spend every Christmas being miserable. This was very hard for me because I *love* Christmas and Christmas music. I was raised believing that Christmas music told the story of the whole meaning of Christmas—and it was a joyful experience—until I married Otis. It never failed; just as Thanksgiving came around, it was like a storm was brewing. Otis would be in the foulest mood. I was scared to even talk to him! I always had to be careful what I said or did for fear he would turn on me. Then, if I was quiet because I was being cautious not to rock the boat, he would holler at me, "What's wrong with you, why aren't you talking to me?!" If I talked to him, I got in trouble. If I didn't, I also got in trouble. It made me feel crazy!

I never had a Christmas with Otis without a heated argument or his silent treatment. I can still recall all the bickering from the moment he or I got home until bedtime and how scary he got. When he scolded me and got in my face, I never felt safe—I was always afraid he was going to hit me. I felt so intimidated and so oppressed when he would tell me, "Shut up, woman!" One Christmas day, I got up early to fix our Christmas meal. I turned on the mini TV in our kitchen to hear the news—at low volume. Evidently, some Christmas music played either through a commercial or perhaps the morning show newscast. I had no clue that it had come on because I was in the middle of reading recipes and cooking. Otis blasted into the kitchen and accused me of deliberately playing Christmas music to annoy him; he said I had no respect for him and started throwing the ingredients I had set out on the counter. When I returned from overseas, Otis had gotten me a kitty cat as a welcome home gift. I had always wanted a cat. Otis not only made a mess that I had to pick up, but then, he also *kicked the kitty* and said we needed to take him back to the store because I had put a red ribbon on its neck, and it was always in his way anyway! Otis left and didn't come back that Christmas night. Otis came back the next morning and showed up at my job apologizing and begging my forgiveness. I didn't want to make a scene so I didn't ask him where he had been. Otis wanted to be forgiven but wouldn't offer up where he had spent the night; if I asked, I knew he would fly off the handle.

Recently, I had seen something on the news that had stayed with me (about the signs of abuse). They had given a hotline phone number to call for more information. I called that number during my lunch break; I told the lady that answered that I thought that I *might* be in an abusive relationship. She asked me a lot of questions, just as if I was filling out some kind of application or something. She asked me if I had a support group, anyone I could call on, that I could count on to help me. I told her that I had called my mama once and that she had said that I had to do my best to work things out because divorce was not an option in our family or the Catholic Church. The lady kept asking me if I felt safe or if I thought that I was in danger. I could never answer the question about feeling safe because for the first time, I realized that I had *never* felt safe when Otis scolded me or when he was out having affairs. I had to admit the truth to myself. That

CASSANDRE'S STORY

Otis had never been my protector—and that hurt me deeply. It wasn't about this last incident, where my safety was threatened. I had to face that even in between those loving, good times, I was *scared* of Otis.

The lady over the phone was very gentle and kind in her soft-spoken voice. She said that if I didn't feel safe, then I had a place to go to which she could arrange to have me stay at. She told me about the women's shelter and that it would all be strictly between her and me—*confidential*. She said all I had to do when Otis left the house was to call the police and that they would escort me to the women's shelter. That same day, before Otis got home from work, I did what she instructed me to do; I packed an overnight bag, put all of my important papers in it, and hid it. Otis was in a fantastic mood when he got home that evening; he even offered to take me out to eat instead of me cooking. I took him up on it. But, things deteriorated after he began to flirt with a few college girls that were sitting in the booth across from us; he even flirted with our waitress. When I confronted him, he said, "Baby, you're just jealous of them. That's what your problem is with other women; it always has been!" Otis actually *denied* his excessive interaction with them and the lack of respect for me as his wife; his tone made me feel guilty for bringing it up.

Otis escorted me to our car and slammed the door after I got in. When he got in the driver's seat, he said in a whispering voice, "We could have had a nice dinner, but you ruined it for us." I asked Otis twice about my kitty cat when we got home because it had disappeared from our apartment. I had gone to the pet store, and they said he hadn't brought it back to them. Otis totally lost it then! Otis started throwing the couch pillows at me and said, "Now, why can't you just drop the subject or the same is going to happen to you—just like your kitty cat!" I didn't talk about it anymore. I went to bed; I was *scared to death* of him. Otis was not only intimidating and threatening in his tone, he was a lot taller and more muscular than me. I knew I couldn't take him down even if I tried to defend myself.

The next day after Otis left for work, I called in sick to work. I contacted the police to come to take me to the shelter. I was so frightened by Otis and terribly afraid of what I was about to do—I was leaving Otis for good. I couldn't tell the people at work that I was quitting because it would blow my cover. I had never stooped so low in my life as to not give notice!

Otis' apologies were not good enough for me anymore; I had heard them for eight years. In the process, I had lost anything and everything that ever meant anything to me. I had sacrificed my life for him, and I wasn't willing to do it anymore; he didn't love me back in return—he was *threatening* me instead. A female and male police officer picked me up and drove me to a shelter that appeared to take an eternity to get to! All I remember about the drive was a numb feeling all over my body and the two cops attempting to argue quietly. The guy cop kept saying that they shouldn't be driving me to this shelter because it was a domestic matter and not their business and because the shelter was out of their county line, and they could get in trouble for taking me there. The lady cop kept saying, "She's in danger. We must help her; that's our job—to save lives!"

The shelter was in a renovated Victorian home, and I love old things, away from the city life! But, it was actually roach and rat infested. I'm sure there are nicer shelters, but I ended up in that one because that's the one that had room for me. There were some bad experiences at the shelter. Like going into the gross kitchen; I didn't even want to eat in there. There were also thieves. Someone got into my suitcase and stole my designer clothes; I was just relieved that they didn't steal my important papers! The good things were: There was a *clean* bathtub and bathroom (that night I took a long, hot bath in an old-fashioned bathtub), they had individual and group counseling, and they helped with job leads. They helped me to plan for a safe place to move to after the shelter.

The best experience I had at the shelter was when I was alone one day (because I had cramps and I didn't go to group). I turned the TV on in the family room where I had laid down to rest, and I came upon a channel that had a pastor speaking. I know now that was an evangelist! It was as if he was speaking directly to me. I ended up hysterically bawling. I had so many tears my vision was blurry. I had so much snot running down my nose and in my throat that I was gagging. I got on my knees and repeated the prayer that was said; I asked Jesus to forgive me. I gave my life over to Him because I had made such a mess out of it, and I had nowhere to turn to. I asked for His healing power. I had been dealing with a lack of appetite and had gotten to where even Otis had noticed my rib and hip bones were showing. More hair than usual was left in my brush and my lips were cracking with flaky, dry, peeling skin—I was anorexic. The next day, my appetite suddenly went back to normal; it was like a huge burden was lifted from me, and I was eating healthy again.

The shelter helped me to get pro-bono legal aid, and Otis was served divorce papers. I was able to find a job in upstate New York in a company that hired administrative translators. I speak French, so that was a tremendous blessing! One of the shelter aids helped me to find a room rental. I loved my new job in the suburbs; it was a stepping stone to save money for a fashion design school! I loved the beautiful home that I now lived in—even though I rented a room, I was allowed to use the common areas. I lived in that home for two years. I felt safe and cared for by the elderly woman who was the home owner. She invited me to go to church with her on Wednesdays and Sundays. I got very close to the Lord and made new church friends at Bible studies and fellowship activities. Otis never showed up at court for the divorce hearing. My lawyer said that a lot of abusive men don't show up because if they are questioned, they don't want it to go on record that they are batterers. She said that most of them avoid having to pay alimony or child support, so if they are no-shows, they *think* they're not held accountable.

After the divorce, *I* began to struggle with the sounds of Christmas! I didn't even realize it until I was at work one day. Christmas music was playing, and I suddenly took a tumble *downward* in my heart. I then noticed it at the grocery store and in department stores the next few days that I couldn't handle all the holiday music they were playing. I had to grab my purchase and get out of there! I would change the radio station if Christmas music came on because it made me very sad. I felt depressed all of a sudden whenever I heard the sounds of Christmas. It was at that point that I prayed and asked the Lord to take those horrible Christmas memories with Otis and to please transform them into something good in me. I asked Him to replace those bad memories with His Peace. Today, I can listen to Christmas music with anticipation of joy and thoroughly enjoy Christmas carols even when it's not Christmas!

It's been three years since the divorce. My mama initially rejected my decision to divorce, but she ended up forgiving me, and we're back to having a close mother-daughter relationship. My sisters welcomed me back like a long-lost friend. My past life is like a nightmare that I can't believe really happened to me. It was dark and evil! I learned new words at the shelter; I learned words like, passive-aggressive. I learned that Otis was passive-aggressive toward me, and that's what made it even more difficult for me to figure out—that I was being abused! Otis was mostly a quiet kind of abuser, but his threats were real and powerful and definitely penetrated my mind and my heart. It was just confusing because he would compliment me all the time on my appearance, and then he would be mean to me and wanting sex after telling me that if I gained weight, he was going to trade me off for a new model like I was some kind of car that he could trade in. I now know that his love was all about my outward appearance and that he didn't love anything else about me. If I got in a car crash and became a deformed invalid, I know he would not stay with me and take care of me as he promised in our vows.

Otis did try to manipulate me back into re-marrying him; he called me, and he also sent me a letter with an enclosed page he tore off from some daily devotional that was on "forgiveness." Otis said in the letter that I had to forgive him because he was a sinner like me and that everyone sins every day. And why couldn't I understand that the only reason he repeated the same things that hurt me was because he was a sinner? If God forgave him every day, why couldn't I? Otis said he loved me and threatened to come get me and bring me back to him, where he said I belonged, and that I was a sinner by not forgiving him. I have a protective order, and I ditched my old cellphone number! Otis wants to retire someday from the parcel company so I doubt he's going to violate the protective order and risk smearing his good image with them by trying to threaten me again.

It has taken time to heal. But my life is full of light and potential now; I look forward to getting up in the morning! If it wasn't for my quiet times with the Lord and my church family, I would be as frightened, lost, hurt, and empty as I was while living with Otis. I was so depressed when I got up in the mornings back then. I don't even miss Otis and his control over my life; he was so controlling that he was not only cheap with everything in our household, but he wouldn't even give money to God! If he did, it was just to make an impression. Back then, he would glare at me whenever I would drop something in the offering plate. I no longer have to have his permission to tithe with my own paycheck.

I'm full of life and fulfilled now. I'm not even in a hurry to get into another romantic relationship—I have my whole future ahead of me for that! I'm attending a fashion and design school, and I'm so grateful for that blessing! I have a driver's license now. My only regret is that I allowed Otis to control me and manipulate my life for more years than necessary. I feel privileged to do my life over, and I cherish the safe and peaceful life that I have today.

PART II

OVERCOMER PRINCIPLES

Overcomer Defined

NOW THAT WE HAVE unearthed the true definitions of an abuser and a victim and we have learned how to balance the Spirit, Mind, and Body, we can proceed to uncover the full meaning of becoming an *Overcomer*. Prepare for victory!

Just exactly what *is* an *Overcomer*? Let's talk about that. While working with victims of abuse, I have always elected not to use the term "survivor." The reason for not using the term "survivor" is because I don't believe in working with victims just to help them exist; I want to encourage them to *stop* living a life of abuse—to permanently conquer and have victory over abuse! Dictionary definitions of *survivor* are: "to remain alive or in existence, live on." The synonyms for *survive* are: "ride out," "weather," and "make it through." A victim doesn't just want to weather and ride out her abuse or make it through her trauma—she wants a fixed line of defense.

When I address or speak of those that have recovered from their abuse, I have always used the term *Overcomer*. Definitions of "overcome" are: "to defeat; conquer, to prevail over, surmount, be victorious." Synonyms for overcome are: "stop," and "triumph." The verb (action) forms and noun (person) forms for "overcome" are: "to conquer" (conqueror), "to have victory" (victor), and "to defeat" (defeater).

In addition to dictionary definitions of an *Overcomer* are the biblical definitions of an *Overcomer*, which are also more fitting for a victim who seeks peace and a permanent resolution to her abusive past, present, and future. The biblical definitions of *Overcomer* are filled with *hope* and *promises for restoration* and *peace*. A victim does not have hope—an Overcomer does. The definition of hope includes the happiness and the good to look forward to. The word hope comes from the Greek word *elpis*, which means to anticipate with pleasure, expectation, or confidence. An *Overcomer* can rest securely in her future because she has hope. Moreover, the biblical definitions of *Overcomer* address the conjoint realms of the victim's Spirit, Mind, and Body, which, when balanced, produce peace.

The Bible equips us with examples of how we are to live. It instructs us on how to rise above our circumstances—in order to live victoriously as *Overcomers*. Followers of Christ are called various names, which include believers, little children, Christians, and *Overcomers*. A victim of abuse, as with all of God's children, is invited to have an indivisible union with Christ Himself, and as a result, she can become a partaker of His victorious, divine nature, which includes the reality that He has the power to overcome—He is an *Overcomer*! An *Overcomer* has the power in Christ to thrive, not just survive.

> "These things I have spoken to you, that in Me you may have peace. In the world you will have

tribulation; but be of good cheer, I have overcome the world" (John 16:33).

Christ is not only encouraging the victim to partake in His divinity (Spirit) and everything that Christ represents (His character), but since He is a victor, He's also offering an opportunity for her to partake in His victory as an *Overcomer*. Anyone who is of God is an *Overcomer*! The victim is given an option to accept and receive all of Christ's inheritance once born of God (see Part IV for the definition of being born of God).

> "For whatever is born of God overcomes the world. And this is the victory that has overcome the world—our faith" (1 John 5:4).

> "You are of God, little children, and have overcome them, because He who is in you is greater than he who is in the world" (1 John 4:4).

There is a warning for the victim who aspires to become an *Overcomer*—the world and satan. The world and satan will attempt to confuse and convince the victim into thinking that satan has victory in the world, and therefore she cannot overcome her victimization and that she will die as a victim. The warning is found throughout the Bible and summarized in Revelation 13:7: "It was granted to him to make war with the saints and to overcome them. And authority was given him over every tribe, tongue, and nation." The saints are those born of God, and yes, satan will make war with them. However, the truth is that those born of God *have overcome* satan! Victims can overcome satan in the same way Christ has. Revelation 12:11 reveals that the saints have won the victory by *overcoming* satan: "And they overcame him by the blood of the Lamb and by the word of their testimony, and they did not love their lives to the death."

When the Bible uses the word "overcome" in Scripture, it translates to listen and hear God's voice, then follow that voice in obedience, reverence, and perseverance. The biblical definition of *Overcomer* means to endure to the end, in spite of suffering, oppression, and rejection. A synonym for *endure* is to cope with. We are to endure to the end because Christ calls us to overcome even our own death.

> "For we have become partakers of Christ if we hold the beginning of our confidence steadfast to the end, while it is said: 'Today, if you will hear His voice, Do not harden your hearts as in the rebellion'" (Hebrews 3:14-15).

> "Now therefore, listen to me, *my* children, For blessed *are those who* keep my ways. Hear instruction and be wise, And do not disdain *it*. Blessed is the man who listens to me, Watching daily at my gates, Waiting at the posts of my doors. For whoever finds me finds life, And obtains favor from the LORD; But he who sins against me wrongs his own soul; All those who hate me love death" (Proverbs 8:32-36).

As an *Overcomer*, the victim learns that it's not about dwelling on her *shame* and the sufferings of her abuse. It's about separating herself from her painful shame because shame is not equal to herself as a person. Pain and shame are a part of the dehumanizing trauma of abuse, which is separate from her dignity and her body as a valued, worthy person. A victim stops at pain; an *Overcomer* parks at peace. She's instead invited to move out of

OVERCOMER PRINCIPLES

pain and shame and to approach God's throne of grace. That's the place to dwell in daily with *perseverance*, just by confidently and boldly coming to His throne. She's to dwell on the prospect of her Spirit *never* dying and receiving a new body as a new creature in Christ, both now and eternally where she will be seated as a royal daughter side-by-side with King Jesus in His Kingdom!

> "Let us therefore come boldly to the throne of grace that we may obtain mercy and find grace to help in time of need" (Hebrews 4:16).

> "To him who overcomes I will grant to sit with Me on My throne, as I also overcame and sat down with My Father on His throne" (Revelation 3:21).

It is *Christ* Who calls the victim to become an *Overcomer*, just like Christ calls each one of us to overcome. An *Overcomer* is promised that she can overcome her troubles with Earth, satan, and hell; she's offered the joy of Christ in her heart and eternal life with Christ in heaven—to be in God's presence—in Paradise. This is undeniably expressed in the Book of Revelation:

> "To him who overcomes I will give to eat from the tree of life, which is in the midst of the Paradise of God" (Revelation 2:7).

> "He who overcomes shall be clothed in white garments, and I will not blot out his name from the Book of Life; but I will confess his name before my Father and before His angels" (Revelation 3:5).

Clothed in white garments? What is *that* all about? The white garments represent purity, holiness, and righteousness with

God. When Christ returns for *all* of the *Overcomers*, they will be clothed in white. That's Christ's color. *Overcomers* will be clothed in Christ's very own holiness and glory. Once an *Overcomer* is born of God, He will not blot out her name from the Book of Life; the *Overcomer* is secure in Christ eternally. When the *Overcomer* arrives in heaven, He will have her crown of life waiting for her. Christ will lovingly welcome her and say, "Father, _____ is home." He may even add a jewel to your crown of life and share a merit tidbit about you as an *Overcomer*, recognizing how proud He is of you, such as when He was introduced by His Father: "This is My beloved Son, in whom I am well pleased" (Matthew 3:17). I smile as I wonder what will He say about unique *you*?

Gaining **awareness, insight, knowledge** and **spiritual revelation** on the dynamics of abuse and its consequences are amongst the must-have vitals before a victim can take the first step out of her abusive cycle to become an *Overcomer*. **Awareness** for an *Overcomer* is crucial: A realization that she has little defense as a victim against the abuser's and society's apathy without God's Word (and God is the Word); Wisdom, Will, and the Supernatural Power of God's favor working through the Holy Spirit within her. **Insight** for an *Overcomer* is absolutely necessary: To know that she needs wisdom, strength, and power beyond herself to end her abusive living. **Knowledge** is imperative: Knowing of the truth that to be an *Overcomer* of abuse, God's *daily* presence is essential in her life. **Spiritual Revelation** is most revelant: An understanding that she has no lasting power in her decision-making—the *self-control* and *restraint* that she needs in following through with her decisions, if she goes without divine intervention. According to God's Word, where there is no revelation, we cast off restraint (Proverbs 29:18). Our wisdom comes from God's revelations through His Word. Our obedience to what He reveals is our choice. He reminds us just the same—that divine obedience brings peace, joy, hope, and blessings!

A victim who has endured the vicious cycle of abuse and has reached rock bottom in her despair is now ready to make a decision to overcome her abuse because the daily darkness is so unbearable, and it overpowers her daily living. She is set to reprogram her victim thoughts into an *Overcomer* mindset. She is at a significant growth point. This stage, although an entrance into the light of freedom from abuse, is a most vulnerable and pressurized state. This is when—regardless of the limited or no support from others, even while too despondent to know what to pray for—she turns all her pain, fears, and concerns over to the One Who is all too aware of what she's been through: Christ. The One Who is her refuge and strength and ever present help in trouble *is* the very One to turn to as her *Overcomer* lifeline.

He has been standing by her side, always ready and willing to provide for her needs. She just has to *ask* for His leadership. This is her cue, the part where she needs to allow Him to be the One to lead her. He will speak to her through His Word and guide her to her next steps, and He will provide His comfort, love, and peace, no matter what the darkest days surrounding her bring. The *Overcomer's* life now overflows with *Overcomer* thinking—and all is derived from setting her focus on an *Overcomer* God—Christ the *Overcomer*! And she will fly, yes, she will fly. His Word says that she will mount up with wings like an eagle (Isaiah 40:31). This means that because she has discovered her purpose in Him, she can now be free to spread her wings like an eagle. Isaiah 40:29 says that He gives power to the weak, and to those who have no might, He increases their strength. She can now fly strong in His Spiritual freedom with clear-sightedness because dark weakness is no longer holding her down!

As a victim, you will have scoffers who will allege that you're using Christianity as a crutch, but they're the ones on a crutch.

The biggest crutch is used by those who are living an unfulfilled, blinded life. They are crippled by their unbelief while you're reaching out to living a faith-filled, fulfilled life. Beware of satan, whose name is also devil, which means *accuser, slanderer, adversary,* or *enemy.* Many in our society have undermined satan's existence and made satan out to be a legendary mythological entity, but he is very *real* just like humans are. The threat and interference of satan is a reality of life. satan is a toxic, poisonous snake—a spiritual terrorist. Jesus Himself had to overcome him (Matthew 4:1-11); such is the case for mankind. satan is neither Jesus' nor your compadre. satan goes around tempting humans so that he can then accuse them before God; he aims to destroy people's lives. The upside is that we don't have to focus on satan's attempts to disrupt our lives, but instead we can opt to redirect our outlook on God's character and Christ's overriding power over satan!

God's eternal power can destroy satan's schemes. God is able to take on his operative militia; satan will never overrule God's purpose or agenda for our lives unless we allow it (God has unconquerable authority over satan's evil forces; satan is powerless over God). satan's resume can't stand up to God's past, present, and future victorious accounts. Don't fall victim to the lies of your accuser, satan, who is not only the greatest accuser but has people whom he uses to prey upon you; he is furious that you belong to Christ and that you are now a part of God's Kingdom (while he is nothing but a fallen dark angel). Keep in mind that satan likes to make you think that he's privy to information about you. Yes, he can watch your actions, he knows about your sin and how he can tempt you into sin, and can interject his thoughts; but he doesn't have the ability to read your thoughts (mind)—only God can do that. God knows everything about everything. satan does not.

OVERCOMER PRINCIPLES

As an *Overcomer*, you are not to be defined by lies. You shall not allow your abuser, nor your accuser, satan, to define you. You are not to define yourself or allow others to define you by what has happened to you or the choices you have had to make. As an *Overcomer*, the only truth about your identity is that you're defined by who you have become in Christ. So, be stamped with Christ's nature as an *Overcomer*! You will then begin to experience His overflowing grace, love, kindness, gentleness, and peace. You will gradually acquire His characteristics and eventually exuberate with His joy and ooze with His humility. satan will do whatever it takes to scare you away from your God-ordained *Overcomer* position. You are loveable, valuable, and precious in God's sight. You will become who Christ says that you are!

I reiterate, when you hear whispers or echoes telling you to go in the direction that will not be safe or ultimately hurt you, that's satan speaking *lies* to you. satan's native tongue is called the language of lying, for he speaks lies as he is the father of lies (John 8:44). Whenever you sense deception, you can be sure he is actively at work. When God is at work in your life, He leads you to the knowledge of *truth* in your circumstances. Becoming an *Overcomer* means letting go of deception and not being a victim who always learns but is never able to move forward in acknowledging the truth about her abusive relationship. satan's onslaught strategy for the victim is that she will become ineffective (the same goal the abuser has for the victim) and never meet Christ and thus have no testimony; or, if she knows Him, his evil schemes plan for the victim's testimony to be ruined. However, an *Overcomer* always has a testimony. If satan attempts to rob you of your *Overcomer* status by whispering that you are anything less than the apple of God's eye, you bind satan and tell him to *get away* and that you are an *Overcomer*! satan will flee because he knows that God can and will restore your victim dignity; satan knows your *Overcomer* status is secure. A victim's refrain must be this: "In the world, I will have tribulation, but I will fear not because my Savior has *overcome* the world!" God is your filter because, He, the Creator of the universe, is your Father—your Daddy—your Protector. He's not going to let you down!

How Does a Victim Become an *Overcomer*?
(1) *Die to self.* When Christ calls a victim to overcome, He first calls her to enter into the knowledge of his profound, unconditional love, followed by a calling to enter into His death encounter. To enter into the circumstances of Jesus' death means to *die to the self* (just as He did in obedience to His Father). She has to die to her *old self* as a person and to separate from and give up the world. It means to give up her personal, worldly plans for her life and to commit to solely living for Him. Any lack of faith (doubt) in the victim's heart or loyalty to past sin is a barrier to fully accepting His love and loving Him in return. It is a resistance to the dying of the old self as a person and as a victim. A victim has to accept Christ's love *fully*, within, or it's impossible to enter into and relate to His death on the cross. Without entering into His unspeakable death experience, Christ cannot live within; the victim cannot accept His love to its fullest because her carnal self continues to be an aversion to God. Listen as Paul and Jesus speak to us in the Bible:

> "I have been crucified with Christ and I no longer live; it is no longer I who live, but Christ lives in me; and the *life* which I now live in the flesh I live by faith in the Son of God, who loved me and gave Himself for me" (Galatians 2:20).

> "Then He said to *them* all, 'If anyone desires to come after Me, let him deny himself, and take up

his cross daily, and follow Me. For whoever desires to save his life will lose it, but whoever loses his life for my sake will save it. For what profit is it to a man if he gains the whole world, and is himself destroyed or lost?'" (Luke 9:23-25).

An *Overcomer* has to use an effortful approach; it is about modification of past emotional memories, healing from unnecessary trauma, saying goodbye to the old self, and rewiring her brain by changing into a new acceptable self. When a victim is captivated by Christ's love, she is enraptured by His love: her entire perspective on life changes. She is able to envision overcoming her abuse through His love as He becomes her hope and her peace. *His* vision and purpose for her life becomes her priority. She is now willing to be obedient to His calling for her as an *Overcomer*: to *live* for Him!

(2) *Love Christ.* Love Him back as *He first* loved you. Christ wants to move with you from head knowledge to *heart* experience. Christ wants to live within you in your heart, where His Spirit resides. *Without* loving Christ, it is *impossible* to overcome anything. Once you accept Christ in your heart, you are bonded in love with Him. You are inseparably linked to Christ's love and presence. This wildly unimaginable gift of love binds you in a spiritual union with Christ that is inseparable and ever after. A victim must realize that accepting Christ's love causes a movement within her and others. An *Overcomer* dwells in the Spirit of His love—the Spirit of *change*. God, Christ, and the Holy Spirit are love—agents of change. For those victims whose hearts are in the God of Christ—who believe in the impossible and *want* to change—change is possible.

"'You shall love the LORD your God with all your heart, with all your soul, and with all your mind'" (Matthew 22:37).

"We love Him because He first loved us" (1 John 4:19).

"Who shall separate us from the love of Christ? *Shall* tribulation, or distress, or persecution, or famine, or nakedness, or peril, or sword?...For I am persuaded that neither death nor life, nor angels nor principalities nor powers, nor things present nor things to come, nor height nor depth, nor any other created thing, shall be able to separate us from the love of God which is in Christ Jesus our Lord" (Romans 8:35, 38-39)

"But He said, 'The things which are impossible with men are possible with God'" (Luke 18:27).

Some victims' measure of worth and love are all tied up with human relationships. In Matthew 10:34-39, Matthew 16:25-26, Luke 14:26-27, 33, God calls us to stop idolizing and following human relationships (friends, family, spouses) and to renounce and exchange the love of these temporal worldly relationships and commodities for a supreme eternal relationship with Him. He is not asking for any unconditional love action toward Him that He hasn't already expressed and demonstrated toward us. He asks that we love Him without conditions and to declare Him as sufficient (as enough)—and to follow Him! Christ states that whoever loves and prefers a human relationship out in the world over a relationship with Him and His Kingdom is not worthy of Him. When a victim is being abused by a natural human relationship she has a choice to prioritize the human relationship or her divine supreme relationship with Christ. She has to ask herself if God is enough, if she is content and satisfied with only His love; and if she's willing to lose a broken human relationship and whatever material possessions, to gain the wholeness Christ? Others may see this as a radical foolish option to choose from but God calls it a wise choice and an exchange for an eternal supreme love—because He is love— like no other love.

(3) *Believe that Jesus is the Christ*. An *Overcomer* must believe that Christ is Lord of Lords, King of Kings, our Savior, Redeemer, and the truth of revelation. An *Overcomer* sees Christ with eyes of faith. When a victim places her faith and trust in the living Christ, it is through Him that she overcomes the danger and adversity that has engulfed her. A victim born of God must not enter into dogmatism, legalism, or religiosity by simply attaining an intellectual understanding of Christ; she must have a surrendered acceptance of the meaning of being born of God and *Who* Jesus Christ *is*. She must *believe* that Christ is who He says He is. The foundation of an *Overcomer* is that she believes in Christ. In Christ, hope is real and alive—hope has another name: Jesus Christ. It is totally about having faith, the kind of faith that overcomes the world! An *Overcomer* has to believe that Jesus *is* God in three persons and that He was crucified by sinners (us) and died for our sins. Becoming an *Overcomer* means surrendering and dedicating her lifetime to Him in love and sacrifice, serving Him as her personal Lord and Savior. Surrendering can only be done by those who are born of God, believe, and want to be *Overcomers*.

There are victims who struggle in their trust to believe, yet they want answers and solutions to their pain. Christ offers victory over satan's tribulations of this world. Even victory over death! All He asks is that you believe that He is God who became flesh and died for your sins and rose again for you. By having faith in Christ, you are born into and granted a new, victorious life, free of being victimized by satan. An *Overcomer* believes, trusts, and readily notices the Hand of God in her life. In order to become an *Overcomer,* you must give up your lack of trust. Trust in Him through faith—that is the ultimate trait of an *Overcomer!* A victim's life is ruled by fear. If you will just trust Him, He will provide renewed overcomer courage for each day. When an *Overcomer* believes and trusts God, she experiences the effervescent life and all of the Holy Spirit's properties which Christ longs to give her. Your time here on Earth is to be lived sight unseen by faith, and heaven is for sight; you as an *Overcomer* will see all that you have been trusting and believing in when you get to heaven.

> "And the Father Himself, who sent Me, has testified of Me. You have neither heard His voice at any time, nor seen His form. But you do not have His word abiding in you, because whom He sent, Him you do not believe" (John 5:37-38).

> "Now faith is the substance of things hoped for, the evidence of things not seen" (Hebrews 11:1).

> "That if you confess with your mouth the Lord Jesus and believe in your heart that God has raised Him from the dead, you will be saved" (Romans 10:9).

> "And those who know Your name will put their trust in You; For You, Lord, have not forsaken those who seek You" (Psalm 9:10).

OVERCOMER PRINCIPLES

(4) *Christ comes first*. Becoming an *Overcomer* means Christ the Lord Almighty comes first—not the world. He *is* the inspirer and designer for each day. An *Overcomer* looks toward the highest power first: Christ. Turning toward anything else first is regarding that object or person as the highest in her life. Facing Christ first will always result in having a communicative relationship with Him and obtaining His feedback on His perfect Will for her life. It is an *everyday* commitment to be an *Overcomer*. It's not about entering into His love and death experience every once in a while—it's a *daily* lifetime commitment. When an *Overcomer* understands that Christ is her priority and accepts His leadership, she can then begin to experience His peace by approaching His throne, no matter what circumstances arise in her new life. The victim does not need a special invitation once born of God; she is encouraged to approach His throne of grace, hope, power, and peace as an *Overcomer* every day. By approaching His throne daily, the victim is transformed into the likeness of Christ (the Holy Spirit's power comes upon and within her).

Deciding to overcome your abuse gives you a life-changing encounter with the One Who will become first in your life. Placing Him first supplies you with a transformation into a life of meaning with a satisfying purpose and complete fulfillment. Putting Christ first requires you to surrender your own will by allowing Him to be the One and only center of your life. Together with Him, you will be able to carry out His will that you live the satisfying, abundant life which He offers. When your eyes are fixed on Christ, He will always come to the forefront, and you'll find that He *is all* and in *all*! We are to be conformed to His Image—not the world's. This is God's eternal Will, that the victim and *all* of His creation will be made into His image. To become like Him requires a renewing of the mind. The *Overcomer* now sees with the eyes of her Spirit; she keeps her inner spiritual vision clear. She's now open to God on the inside, which leads to the renewal of her mind. To become Christ-like, she has to prioritize spending time in His Word so that she may have victory over temptations, tribulations, and endure the world—like Christ has—*as an Overcomer!*

> "But seek first the kingdom of God and His righteousness, and all these things shall be added to you" (Matthew 6:33).

> "And do not be conformed to this world, but be transformed by the renewing of your mind, that you may prove what *is* that good and acceptable and perfect will of God" (Romans 12:2).

> "For whom He foreknew, He also predestined *to be* conformed to the image of His Son" (Romans 8:29).

Once you choose Christ to be first in your life, He will give you the *power* to follow His Spirit, obey His commands, and to accept His eternal, graceful, and merciful forgiveness. Being an *Overcomer* is an inside job! Becoming an *Overcomer* for life must be done through a change in the Spirit and Mind from the inside out; then it manifests itself in the fruit of your Body through your conversion and transformation of actions. Becoming an *Overcomer* is like attending His Spiritual prep school. His Word is your textbook; God the Father, Christ, and His followers are your teachers, mentors, and friends; and the Holy Spirit is your personal coach, trainer, instructor, and assistant.

Victims live an inconsistent life of only being able to display their real self when they feel safe. Sometimes they have to change costumes depending on whether they are at work or around strangers, friends, family, or the abuser. The lifeblood

OVERCOMER PRINCIPLES

of being an *Overcomer* is that everything the victim has become on the inside is now obvious from the outside. An *Overcomer* can feel the Holy Spirit's presence changing her from the inside out as she has removed herself from the world and into Christ's inner circle! There is wholeness about moving from the divided victim role into the complete *Overcomer* person, which means living life from the inside-out and thereby not allowing outside victim triggers to influence the consistency of walking in the protected life of an *Overcomer*.

An *Overcomer* has principles that she abides by; she remains true to her principles, does not suppress her *Overcomer* ideals, and does not bow to the societal pressures to remain a victim. She knows that if she curtsies to that, she is now violating her Christ-ordained character. An *Overcomer* uses mindfulness in balancing her Spirit, Mind, and Body. She has developed a Spiritual consciousness in her mind, knowing that Christ's presence is at work in her through the Holy Spirit; she's now able to interpret the abuse from His perspective instead of from the perspective of her abuser and society. She has learned that what she believes about herself and others is central to her achievement of true peace and freedom in her life. She realizes that she must remain true to only God and herself, even if she is scorned and rejected by many; but in her new, exchanged life, she will partake in the joy and satisfaction of not living a double life.

Amongst the many *Overcomer* rewards, she reaps the knowledge that when she actively pleases God with fervor rather than pleasing her abuser and society, she's able to enjoy a quality of life and happiness compared to none before. When Christ comes first, He resets the *Overcomer*'s priorities in an order that she would not have even begun to think about! She begins to look forward to those new priorities as they become nutritious in her Spirit; she now even welcomes them into her life with wonder and joyful anticipation. When the living Christ within you is first in your life, there can be no argument against the divine positive influence He has in yours and the lives of others whom you impact! Having left her ever-changing world of abuse, an overcomer now has Christ's stability in her life. She no longer lives a daily TBD (to be determined) life based on her abuser's terms for the relationship. Peruse through all of the *Overcomer* principles that have been discussed. Is there any reason why you wouldn't be interested in incorporating them into your life?

To become an *Overcomer* means to disarm the victim mentality. When you give up your victim role, God creates a brand-new road map for you—with freshly inscribed directions—leading you to the best route to take (all the while watching over you and keeping you from harm's way). In order to obtain your new roadmap, you must actively walk your feet in His lighted direction with the *Overcomer* vision He has given you. You must not be afraid of this *Overcomer* journey which seems off the map. God is all-knowing; what is unknown to us is already known to Him. He promises to be your personal Bodyguard as you venture into what appears as an uncharted course. "Your ears shall hear a word behind you, saying, 'This *is* the way, walk in it,' Whenever you turn to the right hand Or whenever you turn to the left" (Isaiah 30:21). Taking the course of an *Overcomer* means relying on what appears to be an obscure beginning but believing in reliable end results.

In Revelation 22:13 God says, "I am the Alpha and the Omega, *the* Beginning and *the* End, the First and the Last." An *Overcomer* knows that Christ is in first place, at center, and last; and that it is only through Christ taking precedence in the heart that a human can reach their highest point in life. An undivided devotion to Christ means not being influenced or dominated (snared) by any created worldly thing; it means complete freedom to be oneself in Christ. One of the most powerful tools that an *Overcomer* keeps in her divine toolbox is her ability to empower herself

OVERCOMER PRINCIPLES

through the Holy Spirit by being determined to challenge any other voice that attempts to derail her belief in Christ, her renewed belief in herself, and her *Overcomer* principles. An *Overcomer* is like a mountain during a snowfall, allowing the snow to drift and melt down without being carried off course. *Overcomers* face an uncertain future with the certainty of a loving Father taking care of what is yet to come. However dark the path ahead may seem, the outcome is that when you're an *Overcomer,* you can look forward to a legacy of a life well-lived! He has paved the way. To become an *Overcomer* is not an unreachable, pious dream; through Christ and the Holy Spirit's help, it is an obtainable goal. The outgrowth from surrendering your victim role is a purging of your brokenness by letting go of your self-will and emerging into being transformed as an *Overcomer*. The outcome is living a life of peace because the sublime peace of Christ *is* the foundation of an *Overcomer's* life. Daughter of God, you can do this! He is ready for you. Are *you* ready?

What to do? What to do? Shall I become an *Overcomer*? Be an *Overcomer*! To *be* is more important than to *do* because you can't be effective in doing without first being. Living a victim life of uncertainty taints your future. When you choose to be an *Overcomer,* your future readily unfolds before you in all its promising confidence. There is no ideal day for you to leave your victim role and to become an *Overcomer*—today is that day! Choosing an *Overcomer* life is a purposeful resolve, or it does not happen. An *Overcomer* operates her lifestyle from the lens of God. She maintains an attitude of confidence and faces the future with expectation. Be an *Overcomer*—you will be clothed with the garment of Peace, what do you have to lose?!

Because of today's corporate calling, which ignores the victim's plight, it requires that the victim become an *Overcomer*, and for her to stand tenaciously firm against settling for society's indoctrinated, misunderstood characteristics of a victim.

However, if you decide to decline Christ's *Overcomer* invitation, know that my heart is sincere when I invite you to consider all that you have read about victimization and to use that information to improve upon your life of abuse.

Overcoming Abuse is a Choice
Leaving the victim role means leaving the world of confusion and foggy thinking that the abuser would like to maintain in the victim's life. As the abuser's love vows conflict with his abusive nature and his ability to convince others that he is *not* abusive, the victim's confusion intensifies as she is already suffocating from his control. Learning to recognize the core dynamics and characteristics of an abuser is the bridge from a victim's state of confusion to an *Overcomer's* clear, objective thinking. An *Overcomer* is able to tell her abuser what's what—simply by taking action on her abuse. *Overcomers* are super-victors; they come out of their sufferance with undaunted radiance, making their victimization totally impotent.

As you've noticed, there are stories of victims who have become *Overcomers* at the conclusions of each part of this book. Have you noticed any abuser, victim, or *Overcomer* characteristics in their stories? Their stories all have an *Overcomer* ending. What is your story? How will your story end? These anecdotes represent a small sample of hundreds of brave victims that I have known who have made a choice to overcome their abuse. These are women who realized that, not only had their *abusers* deceived them, but that they had also deceived their own selves and had become their own prison wardens. This realization brings a breakthrough for a victim, which leads her to admit her abuse to herself and trusted others. All at once, she's able to see new choices for her life despite her painful losses through abuse. She's able to discern that mourning the loss of her dreams and hopes for her marriage does not mean she's mourning the loss of her abuser or abusive lifestyle. She discovers that with some assistance—some mindful thinking and actions—she can release herself from her imprisonment. Becoming an *Overcomer* is a priority decision—it is a life-choice.

She can now rewrite her *victim script* into an *Overcomer script*, a script that takes her in a new direction with the choice of an abuse-free life. The *Overcomer* has learned to now recoil whenever anyone attempts to treat her with vile disrespect! All of her new insights empower her into a *new* view of herself and life—she begins working to overcome her abuse—thereby changing her life *forever*. Some *Overcomers* remain single by choice; others remarry into abuse-free marriages. Just as there are certain terms drawn up for divorce, there are also written terms for some marriages. Prenuptial agreements are not just for the fair and adequate distribution of a couple's assets, but they can also be drawn up for the purpose of agreeing on protection and safety in the marriage. Some *Overcomers* discuss and draw up their prenuptial agreements during their pre-marital sessions, which are usually conducted by their clergy or other professional. The prenuptial agreement clearly states both what the former victim (engaged *Overcomer*) expects regarding respect, protection, and safety and what she will *not* tolerate (itemized abuse tactics) in the marriage. It is clearly stipulated that in the event that the prenuptial agreement is violated, she is free to end the marriage.

Post-Escape Safety Plan
Before reading this section, bow your head down, close your eyes, and pray to God; thank Him for having given you His protection through His Spirit and the assistance of many during your journey out of your abusive home. Praise Him for having granted you safe passage and for delivering you out of your evil and dangerous circumstance. Give the glory to Him for helping you and for making it possible for you to escape your abuse.

Thank Him in advance for His continued protection of you. "But Jesus looked at *them* and said to them, 'With men this is impossible, but with God all things are possible'" (Matthew 19:26).

Having graduated from the level of working through a Safety Escape Plan while living with the abuser, and having separated from him, a victim is now ready to implement a Post-Escape Safety Plan (PESP). The following are some post-escape safety strategies which are not limited to this list, but rather, have to be tailored to the new Overcomer's circumstances:

1. Before you move out of your safety resource, secure an *updated* protection order on your abuser. Make multiple copies of the protection order and keep them on your person and everywhere you go (school, work, church, gym).
2. Never walk or drive the identical routes when you travel to your places of commitment.
3. Notify your county police, your neighbors, employer, co-workers, and children's school of your abuser's danger status, and provide a photo of him along with a description of the vehicle(s) he drives.
4. Have an established safety plan that if your abuser approaches your children that they will *not* speak to him. Ask them to seek the agreed upon resources for help. Provide prepaid phones for your older children and instruct them to call 911 if the abuser shows up.
5. Secure an established safety protection plan with your local police should your abuser violate your protection order.

Having a well-developed PESP will provide you with confidence and reassured security. If you stay in your home, the only way you will feel safe (even if you have a restraining order) is if you change your door locks and have a security system installed which prompts you to alert the police if your abuser shows up on your property. If you left with a vehicle in your name, be

OVERCOMER PRINCIPLES

sure to change the door locks in your car. Be grateful for that new chance at life and the new journey that you will begin as an *Overcomer*. An attitude of gratitude for your new abuse-free life can help to pull you out of your trauma of abuse. Your abuser may have been a huge stumbling block in your life, but God will work it out so that your abuser is just a past pebble and is now a stepping stone into living your life as an *Overcomer*. An *Overcomer* places God first over the abuser, lets go of the abuser's intimidating tactics, and is able to be on the offensive, encouraging herself, knowing her God, His guidance, her support system, and *Overcomer* lifestyle will bring her out of captivity. "*We are* hard-pressed on every side, yet not crushed; *we are* perplexed, but not in despair; persecuted, but not forsaken; struck down, but not destroyed" (2 Corinthians 4:8-9).

Sometime your abuser may come back. Even if he is or you are involved in another relationship, engaged, or remarried, this does not matter to him. Research shows that the abuser doesn't change his abuse toward the victim once she terminates the relationship. Your abuser may attempt to wield you back into the relationship during your "end state." This is a time to stay strong. Research from The National Domestic Violence Hotline shows that the average victim leaves her abuser seven times before she leaves him permanently. During the end-cycle of abuse, some victims separate, return, renew their vows, divorce their abuser, reconcile, and remarry the abuser before the final departure. It is preemptive that a victim gets past the separation step and applies her *Overcomer* principles as a daily practice if she's not going to be controlled by the abuser after leaving him.

Your abuser can slip back into your life before you even know that it is happening. Your abuser will contact you at your weakest moment. An abuser knows to contact his victim when she's stressed from work, ill, having problems, or facing an upcoming emotional family event (wedding, funeral) because he can play into the victim's vulnerable state. Your abuser will underhandedly coerce you with his purported changed person and will love-bomb you back into his life. Yes, *his* life, because with an abuser, you will no longer have a life of your own. If you attempt to separate your identity from his, he will find a way to indirectly or directly act out and get your attention back to him! This is a good time to think about the positive headway that you have made toward an abuse-free life. Bring to mind how you have thus far successfully navigated through the grief transition. To give you strength in the present, use your new knowledge on how bravely and strongly you coped before when you felt weak. Yes, it appeared too traumatic to deal with the separation, but *Overcomer*, deal with it you did.

Do not allow your mind to migrate back to the abuser and how good it would be if he changed. Such a thought is part of the grieving process for a victim of abuse. Though this has been an unthinkable loss for you, trust that Christ will take good care of you. If you are haunted by unresolved grief about "what could have been," you will not be able to be set free in your spirit—you won't experience the freedom of peace that is your spiritual heritage. Christ's merciful atonement provides a vision of what you can become. Your past and loss of future plans in the abusive relationship may grieve your heart, but the light of an *Overcomer*'s life supersedes the unpromising dark past. As an *Overcomer*, you have a daily spiritual opportunity to begin anew with God—fully undisturbed by sorrowful thoughts of poor choices, past failures, or losses. An *Overcomer* lives with an underlying peace in her heart.

An abuser doesn't randomly stop abusing; he just changes his approach and format as to *how* and through *who* or *what* he attempts to abuse in order to re-victimize the *Overcomer*. Your abuser does this to threaten your safety and to be a killjoy; he wants to assert his dominance and control by attempting to scare you and steal every ounce of your joy. Remember God's command is for you to remain faithful not fearful; with His presence, there is no room for fear. Fear is not from God (2 Timothy 1:7). Never surrender to fear. The command to "be strong and courageous" appears over ten times in the Bible for a reason. God knows your fears and what your abuser is capable of. Not to worry, through His Spirit He is right there with you; your Heavenly Father sees *everything* that's going on. The Holy Spirit can free your heart and your mind from fear; He can restore your joy. *He* is your joy, and your joy cannot be stolen unless you allow it to be. "Have I not commanded you? Be strong and of good courage; do not be afraid, nor be dismayed, for the Lord your God *is* with you wherever you go" (Joshua 1:9); "The name of the Lord *is* a strong tower; The righteous run to it and are safe" (Proverbs 18:10). Listen to God's voice of Truth which says, "Be strong and courageous!"

It's sometimes impossible for some victims to discipline themselves into reading God's Word while they're undergoing so much pain because concentration is very difficult; their frightened thoughts take over, those thoughts keep returning to their pain, and the fear in their circumstances keeps creeping in, making it hard to think or read clearly and stay focused. When you do return to read God's Word, it stimulates your mind, and you will feel His love and presence. His love bleeds and spills over from the pages of His Word to soothe, comfort, and restore you. In the meantime, the exercise below allows an option for staying in the presence of God by strategically focusing on Him during those difficult, painful days.

Every time your abuser comes back to haunt your mind or show up physically, and it becomes too difficult to visualize going forward or too painful to look back on the past, causing you to feel weak, you have to adapt a new perspective, a new vision to focus on. "Set your mind on things above, not on things on the earth" (Colossians 3:2). *Visualize* your Heavenly Father, your strong tower, and *focus* your eyes on Him! Stay the course, and every time you lose your focus and you're distracted with thoughts that are away from Him, repeat the following thought out loud: "Visualizing and focusing on you, Jesus!" If you keep your vision focused on your Heavenly Father, you will be able to bear the past and move forward. Ask yourself, "What is your focus on?" Set a timer, and each time the abuser comes to mind, do a *focus exercise* for a half hour, then increase it to an hour, or longer (you may read His Word, a devotional, watch an inspirational music video, or whatever focuses on *Him*). Some use background instrumental music with nature, forest, or ocean sounds during this exercise. Some like upbeat praise and worship songs. Some prefer silence. One of my patients, in addition to her focus exercise, worked at her computer and listened to praise and worship music in the background in case her abuser would come to mind. If her abuser invaded and intruded her thoughts, she would bring up that minimized window and watch the accompanying inspirational music video. Place *God* as the focus of your attention, making Him the center of your life, and see what happens to you when your focus is totally on Him!

This visual and focus exercise is preferably done by selecting a quiet place to sit still. It must be a time that's technology/social media-free and secure of no interruption from others. Have your Bible, a notebook, or journal with you to write any inspirational thoughts or insights gained. If your thoughts wander away from your focus on Christ, redirect your thoughts back to your focal point. This exercise is similar to what's recommended to alleviate the contraction pains of a woman in labor. She is encouraged to use a focal point and to use all of her energy to look at and think about her focal point during her contraction, thus reducing her level of pain at its highest peak. It's similar to riding a tidal wave when it's coming toward you. You don't just stand still and allow the wave to crash upon you and drown you; you strategically concentrate and focus on riding the wave as you move afloat on top of it! Focus on Him, *run* to Him. You will suddenly find Him, be afloat, and be safe in the presence of His loving Arms wrapped around you!

To feel God's *presence* in your innermost being requires sensitivity to the guidance of the Holy Spirit and a willingness to take a risk by trusting Him completely. You may be struggling with your faith and wavering in your belief that there's even a God because you wonder, "Where is He, and how could He allow this abuse to happen to me?" Turning to Him through this focus exercise will help you to sense His presence, and all it requires is for you to be creatively active in pursuing His nearness. It is an act of courageous faith, but Christ never disappoints those who believe and have faith in Him. If you're hurting so much that your faith is decreasing, remind yourself that God's presence is near, and He promises to empower you even when your faith is as small as a mustard seed. "So Jesus said to them, 'Because of your unbelief; for assuredly, I say to you, if you have faith as a mustard seed, you will say to this mountain, 'Move from here to there,' and it will move; and nothing will be impossible for you" (Matthew 17:20).

You will never be the same each time you complete this focus exercise because the power of the Holy Spirit takes over. When you spend time focusing on God and His truths revealed through Christ within you, it is highly unlikely that you will remain weak and in emotional pain. There is power in focusing on Him through prayer, praise, and worship of Him. The healthiest *Overcomers* you will ever meet are those who choose to take a daily dose of God's presence within them. The challenges from your abusive world become much clearer when you look at them from a higher perspective. At the conclusion of each focus exercise, you'll notice a peace and begin to believe that everything will be alright, that you can *trust* your Heavenly Father, and that you *can* actually do all that you need to do to move forward.

To truly experience God's complete presence while under severe abuse trauma requires a deep level of faith and commitment. Some victims don't believe His presence is attainable while undergoing such fear and duress, but God's Word says otherwise. God says that with Him, *all* things are possible. All that is required is to believe in *faith* and to surrender one's mind to the mind of Christ. The cure for all fear and pain is not about religiosity; it's about knowing Him and committing one's life to His guidance. It is about consciously being aware of His living presence. It is about experiencing the relief from the stressors and His *peace* replacing the fear and pain with His dynamic presence. The victim is no longer a slave to fear but is instead a servant to a Spiritual Master who is within her—to serve *her*—through His divine presence.

If you decide to leave your victim role and accept that the secret to living in freedom is the fact that Christ lives and is present within you, then you have discovered the greatest mystery revealed to you as an *Overcomer*; it is offered to anyone who chooses to live out the dynamics of a Christian lifestyle. This is when your trust is realigned, recognizing that Christ is very much alive in your thoughts and emotions and manifests Himself in your actions. This revelation will carry you through from victimization to the spiritual heights of an *Overcomer* in Christ. All that you used to fear attempting now becomes possible, and the things that used to frighten you no longer scare you. The mysterious secret of Christ's living presence within you and in others around you empowers you to face your *Overcomer* life with peace, confidence, hope, and expectation. You are now under Christ's secure presence; it is not a mystery to you, but maybe it is for others that don't know Christ. Your life has changed because Christ's Spirit now works within you, and you remain secure in Him. If ever victim fear crops up, you thank Him for your freedom from fear and the life of abundant mercy, grace, comfort, peace, and security which He has given you!

Always remember that placing *Christ* first means seeking *God's* wisdom. When your abuser attempts to contact you—turn to God for discernment. *He* has provided you with a body of knowledge and resources that have empowered you out of your victim role—use them! Further, turn to Him not just for His guidance but for His comfort as well because His Word promises, "Blessed *be* the God and Father of our Lord Jesus Christ, the Father of mercies and God of all comfort" (2 Corinthians 1:3). He's Jesus' Father and your Father, too. He's your Maker and offers to be your groom and spouse if you need a husband: "For your Maker *is* your husband" (Isaiah 54:5). *The God of the whole Earth loves you*! If you haven't already asked Him to be your groom, ask Christ today: "Will you forgive me and come into my heart and my life? Will you be my groom?" Once you ask Him into your heart, your soul becomes linked to His heart; the two of you become one, as a bride and groom. Essentially, you are saying back to Him what He has said all along, "Let's do life together." Why wait to pop the question? After all, it is the most important question you will ever ask in your life! Need His mercy? Need His comfort? He's the great "I AM WHO I AM" (Exodus 3:14). He is your safe haven. He's your All-in-All. His love is plentiful. Go to Him!

You can rest assured that He is not only The Great "I AM," but once you commit to Him, you will also be certain to say, "He is the God of all I am!" He has a boundless reservoir of compassion that's available whenever you need it. The Lord picks up a victim or *Overcomer* at whatever phase she's in. He gazes into her eyes with His compassion that runs through His veins; He imbues her with His Spirit of love and direction. He knows that it is possible to be the victor and still have the bruises (trauma) and the aftermath. He will renew and transform you through His unfailing affection. Let Him pick you up and embrace you—He will restore your mood and guide your path. *Overcomer*, you are going to deliberately burn bridges behind you and build new ones ahead of you. Choose safety. HE is your safe, secure foundation!

Overcomer Characteristics

What are the criteria that determine whether a victim has indeed entered into the role of an *Overcomer*? The list that follows indicates some of the characteristics of an *Overcomer*. A victim of abuse would have to have met the following criteria in order to experience healing from abuse; these are indicators that the victim has healed and has indeed become an *Overcomer*:

- She has identified her sense of self and continues to purposely develop and mature neurologically and spiritually.
- She is able to control her own mind and uses brain integration and spiritual wisdom to discern and make decisions. She uses her wise decision-making abilities.
- She feels empowered and able to control the choices that she makes and is actively alert to use good judgment on the situations out of her control.
- She is assertive and confident because she has regained her self-worth.
- She has made amends with friends and family and/or has developed and established new supportive relationships.
- She has conquered or brought her physiological post-traumatic symptoms to manageable limits.
- She can choose to think about her abuse memories, or not, through remembering her trauma or putting it aside.
- She has authority over her feelings regarding her abusive memories whereby she can tolerate the feelings associated with her trauma without experiencing symptoms.

OVERCOMER PRINCIPLES

- She has established safety strategies, has restored her self-respect, and has learned the warning signs of an abuser.
- She has learned to balance the dynamics of dominance and submission in a healthy relational style.
- She has re-written her life story without skipping or blocking portions of her life; her abuse trauma is extrapolated from her victim role and incorporated into her meaningful life experiences as a triumphant *Overcomer*.
- She has found a purpose for her past, present, and future.
- She has reached a balance, knowing total isolation is from satan, and fellowship is from God.
- She embraces her freedom from abuse and actively pursues the same freedom for others.
- She has regained her identity, is experiencing *peace* in the midst of *any* circumstances, and is actively pursuing the development and balance of her Spirit, Mind, and Body.
- She radiates God's love.

An *Overcomer* chooses not to allow her past victim role to define her; she chooses to use her victimization as a learning and training tool for the present and future. *Overcomers* put their overcomer principles into action. It's like they have X-Ray vision, and as they grow, they are able to divinely discern with CAT scan vision. *Overcomers* become wise thinkers in developing their Spirit, Mind, and Body. *Overcomers* no longer avoid facing their circumstances that will have to be faced at some point. The Holy Spirit prompts an *Overcomer* out of spiritual and mindless short-sightedness. *Overcomers* are farsighted; they look out for their lives and their next generations; not just for the present outcome but for the future and eternity. *Overcomers* know Who, what, when, why, how, and where their Power Source comes from—and that it is infinite!

The *Overcomer* Lifestyle
Becoming an *Overcomer* requires having resolved the traumatic past abuse; it's all about creating an abuse-free present and future—*now*. It is only through using maximum exertion of the Spirit and the will that it is possible for the victim to reinstate and claim her new identity as an *Overcomer*. The *Overcomer* has to come to terms with saying a final goodbye to her abusive past life, but before doing so, she has had to grieve the loss of her past self-identity, which was destroyed; and now, she has to greet her new self-identity. I have had victims tell me that restoring their identity was similar to their search to find out who their abuser truly was, that it was like peeling back all the layers of an onion to get to the core of his empty, true identity. They have used the same approach on themselves, which they said felt like having to pull back all the layers of abuse to find the heart of the identity they used to have. Every facet and relationship in an *Overcomer*'s life has been challenged and forever changed by her traumatic abusive past. She has had to bury her past belief system and welcome a new belief system based on eternal faith. She has surrendered her meaningless and purposeless life in the cycle of abuse. Through this resignation of her past, she is able to accept her *new* Spirit and renewed *soul*.

The victim has finally accepted the life of an *Overcomer*; she realizes that she has met up with her Life-Giver. She has new hardwiring that provides a very personal, powerful, and wireless relationship and connection to her God. The Holy Spirit now indwells in her heart. A victim's revelation about the reality of the abusive life she has lived through is marked by an epoch-making discovery of a new stratosphere—an *Overcomer* life that she can now live to its fullest! With her new empowered self, an *Overcomer* can integrate *all* that she has learned from her traumatic experiences into her abuse-free lifestyle. *Overcomer* principles take over and become standard operating procedures. She

OVERCOMER PRINCIPLES

takes steps to exert her healthy ability to assert herself and use a balanced sense of power and control in her life; she's willing to bond with those whom she has elected to trust and to be a part of her life; she has learned many lessons on how to protect herself from spiritually, emotionally, and physically dangerous relationships. The *Overcomer* lives her life with praise and thanksgiving. An *Overcomer* has a transfigured *faith* attitude that is inward, outward, and forward in the present and future.

She has learned to appreciate nature and the little things in life that mean a lot. Her priorities have changed, and she's clear about what's meaningful and what's not. An *Overcomer* manages her time wisely. She not only sets priorities, but she acts on them. She has simplified her life around those priorities. She dreams openly—no longer pushing aside her goals because the shout from abuse was calling for her attention. God has lifted her out of her deepest abyss and has destroyed every abuser tactic that was vying for her attention. She's careful to prioritize the callings from God that are worthy of her attention and time. Having experienced living with evil, she now treasures what is full of goodness. An *Overcomer* rejoices and partakes fully in her newfound life, recognizing along the way what is temporal and unimportant, while celebrating the promises of what's eternal.

An *Overcomer* has learned that the root of her hopelessness stems from her abuser's rejection and refusal of her as an individual with an identity. A victim's hopelessness is only found in her heart, not in her circumstances; an *Overcomer* knows that God has more than enough love, power, and provision to avert abuse. She knows that she no longer wants the attachment or companionship of an abuser who can only live for himself and does not want to share life experiences. An *Overcomer* overcomes the false hope, against all the odds, that someday she will be able to develop and establish a genuine relationship with her abuser. An *Overcomer* no longer needs the nurturing of an abuser who is incapable of being nurturing; she is God-nurtured and has learned how to self-nurture without all of the constraints of an abusive relationship. *Overcomers* develop genuine relationships through which they can talk openly without fear of condemnation. Time and experience have taught the *Overcomer* that longing for genuine communication and a connection is a fruitless effort with an abuser who consistently turns her down in more ways than one.

Overcomers are no longer attracted to abusers who only frustrate and hurt their need for honesty and open interaction. A victim knows when she has conquered her victim role and has now become an *Overcomer* because she no longer allows the abuser or anyone else to discount her as a person; she has found her self-value which has always been there, and she now reaches out to the Lord and herself to advocate for herself and others. *Overcomers* seek and meet persons with the same healthy needs for genuine communication; it's as if the *Overcomer* becomes allergic to toxic, unhealthy contacts that can spark a reaction within her. An *Overcomer* refuses to become overwhelmed and give in to unhealthy contacts or former abusers. An *Overcomer* never gives up her divine, unlimited power which she now has over her renewed unconscious and conscious life. She has learned that she could not live life fully while staying connected to her abuser—without paying for it with depression and safety risks.

A victim comes in on the first rung of the ladder and is usually hesitant, not knowing whether to continue upward, but once placing her foot there, the Spirit of God takes over to comfort, strengthen, balance, and guide her to the top. When an *Overcomer* detaches herself from her abuser, she re-experiences for the first time in a long time the divine and human feeling of warmth, empathy, and freedom from blame and unreasonable demands. Most victims have experienced the feeling of yearning for and expecting something by way of *comfort* but without truly knowing what it was; an *Overcomer* knows now what it's like to have a *Comforter*. She has found the peaceful serenity she used to yearn for through her new Comforter. She can now sense and experience the presence of the Holy Spirit's comfort.

An *Overcomer* doesn't feel controlled by her abusive past; she's in control of her own life. She has an in-depth understanding of the victim that lived within her, of *whom* she used to be, and of the trauma done to her. An *Overcomer* no longer engages in self-damnation and now incorporates *truths* into her life that remove the onus from her. The *Overcomer* is able to understand and accept that the abuse was not about her *performance* in the relationship but about one person—her abuser. *Overcomers* realize that they have a choice for safety, even when encountering some non-supportive attitudes from their peers, family, and society. She—the *Overcomer*—fully comprehends that she is now free to become who she was truly called to be. An *Overcomer* learns that ending the relationship is not the only solution to overcome abuse; it has to be coupled with the re-writing of her life script in order to practice the necessary strength and lifestyle that's required so as to not return to her abuser or move on to yet another abusive relationship.

She is able to clearly reflect on the positive aspects of the person that she was before her abusive relationship, the experience of being abused, and the process of recovery; and, she incorporates all of these to recreate her new fabulous reprogrammed self. An *Overcomer* feels liberated as she steps off the path of abuse and moves forward with her life. She has learned that the direction that she takes in life will determine her fate. Having decided her direction in life, she now feels able to face her own life with a sense of inner joy and tranquility. Sometimes, having peace on a day-to-day basis appears and feels alien to her, as the past has always been full of crisis, and she's had to run on adrenaline all of the time. The more the *Overcomer* engages in recreating her new self and life, the more she will gradually adapt and become tolerant of the abuse trauma memory, the way it used to be, and the way it does *not* have to be. The high level of tolerance for acknowledging the way it *used to be* and the way that *it is now* strengthens the *Overcomer* as she realizes that she now possesses personal and divine adaptive resources that she can use to fulfill her new identity as an autonomous *Overcomer*.

Never again does she as an *Overcomer* have to seek refuge through an abuser; an *Overcomer* is self-assured that *God is there* and that there are persons who are willing and available to comprehend the trauma of abuse. Victims remain trapped in unrealistic, emotionally-inhibited, fairytale-inspired relationships; *Overcomers* free themselves from living in the illusory world of the abused—*Overcomers* recognize the difference. An *Overcomer* comes to terms with the truth that it is futile to believe that the abuser will ultimately become a sincere individual with a caring attitude. She now knows that only the abuser can change his attitude and behavior; only *he* can choose to engage in respectful dialogue. The *Overcomer* no longer lives with the illusion of her abuser changing, and she can easily distinguish the *now* from *back then*. An *Overcomer* does not have to change her self-identity to be accepted by others; she actually takes pleasure in developing relationships with people that look up to her but are not expecting her to be preterhuman. An *Overcomer*'s lifestyle enjoys the fullness of the abundant life; it's a quality of life that is incomparable to the victim's past mere existence. An *Overcomer* is a living monument of God's power!

An *Overcomer* has Purpose
Only God's generous grace, mercy, and power can keep a victim from falling. If she does fall, He simply picks her back up. Most *Overcomers* recover from their abusive past and their role as victims within the perimeters of their own personal redemp-

tive life. An *Overcomer* is redeemed by the Lord. Some are called as a result of their redemptive story to tell others about their past abusive trauma, not just as a call for social action, but as a *mission* of alliance with victims that need to hear that there is hope and everlasting peace to be found in becoming an *Overcomer*. This *Overcomer* calling is not just good encouragement for those that are suffering from the tragedy of abuse, but it also serves as a way for the *Overcomer* to share her spiritually mature and adaptive coping strategies through demonstrating her fruit of the spirit: love, joy, peace, longsuffering, kindness, goodness, faithfulness, gentleness, and self-control (Galatians 5:22-23). An *Overcomer* lifestyle is all but static. By the power of the Holy Spirit, it is filled with life-giving energy, which enables the *Overcomer* to grow into the spiritual maturity that exudes the fruit of the Spirit. At the end of the day (and your life), God is always a purposeful God. I get so excited when I watch as God unfolds an *Overcomer*'s purposeful life!

Participating in a mission to help others that are involved in an abusive relationship is one of the strong key indicators that a victim has overcome her abuse. An *Overcomer* lays the foundation of encouragement for a victim as a pipeline to the development of *Overcomer* goals; it's an indispensable act. *Overcomers* can become conduits of love and encouragement to victims. All *Overcomers* know that encouragement is like oxygen to a victim, that oxygen is the daily breath that enables her to overcome. Helping victims of abuse brings out the best in the *Overcomer*. An *Overcomer* has a hardy spirit; she can kindle and transfer that *Overcomer* hardihood to victims at risk! *Overcomers* come to realize that the abuse that was forced upon them *cannot be undone,* no matter how much they hoped for restitution. Restitution from the suffered abuse—no. Restoration of the self—yes. *Overcomers* realize that it's important to confront the abuser and to hold him accountable for his criminal act of abuse, not only for their own personal well-being, but also for the education, justice, and health of victims and society as a whole.

By sharing her victim and *Overcomer* testimony, the *Overcomer* deters the abuser's attempt to continue isolating her from the public; he cannot maintain her silence as she opens up and finds allies in her community. When members of a community hear someone testify to criminal acts of abuse, they are more open to seeking justice for the members of their community; they understand that the *Overcomer*'s legal battle can benefit others in their community. Each *Overcomer* can bring public awareness regarding spousal abuse; such information can influence educational, legal, and political action to prevent the victimization of others that are involved in marital abuse. If family violence is to be resolved, our country must go beyond proactive measures. Every city and state in the U.S. has a system in place for dealing with what they call "domestic violence," but the reason this system isn't working is because they are big on system (policies and procedures) and small on proactivity that's followed by solution-based action.

It is the *Overcomers* who have the *most* personal experience with the natural human phenomenon of ignoring the atrocities that are inflicted upon victims of abuse. The *Overcomer* may have used this approach herself in her past (as a victim in denial or fear) and realizes now that ignoring only leads to repeating the vicious cycle of abuse. It's the *Overcomer*'s public truth-telling that brings attention to this grievous social problem, which, in turn, can lead to social action, liberating victims and bringing abusers to justice. This is a way that the *Overcomer* can make a purposeful contribution to breaking the cycle of community family violence. In addition, an *Overcomer* can become a channel for God's love and mercy toward the victims of this world.

She can become an ambassadress of redemption for victims of abuse. It only takes the Holy Spirit to embolden an *Overcomer* into sharing with a victim the revived, exciting course in life that she can have if she goes forward with an abuse-free life. There is hope in knowing that deeply transformed victims can experience change in their lives, which can have an impact on those in their environment. Changed victims can change society. With today's technology, changed victims are *Overcomers* that can influence the international world of abuse around them. *Overcomers* can lead society to frontiers that have never been crossed before, and they can successfully change a world of trauma for the better.

> "Though I walk in the midst of trouble, You will revive me;
> You will stretch out Your hand
> Against the wrath of my enemies,
> And Your right hand will save me.
> The LORD will perfect *that which* concerns me;
> Your mercy, O LORD, *endures* forever;
> Do not forsake the works of Your hands."
> Psalm 138: 7-8

GRACE'S STORY

KARL AND I MET in Springfield, Missouri. During that time, young people from the surrounding small towns would drive around the square to meet and greet one another. It was how we hung out; that's how I met Karl. We then talked on the phone and began to date. I was a freshman in college getting my bachelor's degree in religion (he had graduated from high school a couple of years before me). Karl had decided not to go to college; he elected to work as a farmer. We got engaged my junior year, and after my graduation, we got married through the Methodist church that I attended. I accepted salvation at age twelve, and my commitment to my faith was important to me and my family. Karl was from the Apostolic Christian faith but had not declared or made a commitment to his church. Although his parents and the church wanted him to become a member and a part of their church family, Karl wouldn't commit.

    I worked in a human resources facility and continued my education in order to earn my master's degree in psychology. We have four children: two sets of twins. The very first time that I became aware that I was being emotionally abused was after the birth of my first set of twins (during our third year of marriage). It became apparent to me that Karl had withdrawn into not conversing with me—he only talked to me as needed through general conversation. We no longer communicated in relationship to one another, like discussing how our day went. There was just no interest on his behalf. The Karl that I had known was no longer there. Karl was not joking or kidding with me anymore. Karl was not playful; he was no longer talking to me. We were not socially connected.

It dawned on me that I felt like he was married to his work. Karl wasn't animated about *anything* but his work; his focus and interest was his job and there was *no* interest in *me*. Karl's time at home was eating, sleeping, and the brief time that he spent with the kids; he repeated this cycle every day. It was as if we had become two people raising kids and didn't have much of a relationship at all. We no longer had an intimate relationship other than a sexual one—it was just sex. If I approached him about our lack of conversation and intimacy as a couple, the discussion would end up in an argument because he saw anything that I didn't agree with him on as me being argumentative. If I saw things differently than he did, he thought I was arguing with him. Whenever I shared that my feelings were hurt, he would see it as a disagreement, and he would just shut down.

If I mentioned that our marriage needed to be focused on God and that we needed a balance with God first, our marriage and family second, jobs third (which would bring us closer together), Karl just remained uninvolved. That's when I really started realizing that Karl didn't have a personal relationship with God. I had kind of doubted that he had this relationship all along, but this is when it became very clear to me. I asked Karl to have devotional times with me. I wanted to have a prayer life with him, but when I pursued this with him, he would never step up to the plate to be a part of it. Karl would not initiate prayer; he would

GRACE'S STORY

not reciprocate prayer. I was virtually placed in an uncomfortable position of spiritually leading.

Although it was a gradual realization that I was in an abusive relationship, there did come a point where I began to think that I had not seen Karl for what he really was. This emotional abuse experience was new to me because I didn't experience any abuse growing up in my family. My parents and I were close, and they were involved with me. Karl was not physically or sexually abused in his past (that I know of), but with his family religious background beliefs, there may have been some emotional deprivation. I think this because his family's faith believes that they are the only one right denomination. There's an unspoken attitude that they are the chosen ones, and unless you're a member, then you're an outsider—which Karl was. Consequently, Karl's parents didn't have much of an emotional relationship with him. Karl would not talk about his feelings toward his parents. I noticed Karl's parents didn't believe in sports or that kids ought to play sports in school or get involved in extracurricular activities. It was all about the farm, and there was no time or reason for all the extras.

The more that our relationship was neglected, the less of a relationship we had. and the more we weren't getting to where I yearned for our relationship to be. I would think, "This just doesn't seem right!" But, even though I didn't see much hope, I told myself, "I'm going to keep trying and trying." By now, our second set of twins were born. I kept convincing myself that I needed to stay in the marriage, and so I did—for thirty-one years. Karl did agree to marriage counseling when our oldest children were in high school and the youngest in middle school. We saw two different therapists which Karl refused to go back to. The first one he got mad at because she wouldn't read an over twenty-page write up about me; it was filled with his opinionated statements saying that I shouldn't be the way that I was and live the way that I did—especially about our finances and the way *he* thought it should be. Karl was zeroing in on the finances with regards to his having every expense and income to the dollar regarding his farming, whereas he felt I spent too much. In particular, he blamed me for the fact that he didn't want any more children after our first set of twins and that I had wanted to have another child.

I ended up having two more because I had twins again, and he was upset about the things that I thought were important. Karl blamed me and believed we should have stopped when we had two kids and not gone on to have four. Karl put me on the spot as being the one who messed it up because I had these desires and beliefs of my own (that we should have more children). Karl said that I couldn't see the bottom line on the expenses.

Karl didn't want to go back to see the second therapist because he said they wouldn't see eye to eye. Karl thought that she wasn't going to see it *his way*. Karl had barely agreed to go to counseling with me, and when it didn't go *his way*, he didn't want to stick to it; he checked out! Prior to going to therapy with me, Karl hadn't given much credibility to counseling (even though it's my profession). So, after his two attempts, he became anti-therapy, and I felt that he never really gave it a chance.

If I had not pinned Karl down and suggested that we needed to talk so many times and on so many levels, we would still be doing more of the same. There came a last time when I said *one more time*, "I don't think that I can take this anymore." We were simply living under the same roof, sleeping together, yet had no relationship whatsoever. I had told him so many times that I couldn't go on having a one-sided relationship. Neither one of us was happy. The kids were all young adults now, and we had the empty nest. I was forced to look more deeply at myself; this was a turning point for me. Had I not taken the bull by the horns and requested that we talk, our relationship would have never been addressed. Yes, at some point I had been in denial, but I now saw that *yes*, this is really what's happening in our relationship! I wrote a letter to Karl explaining that I was very unhappy and that I couldn't continue in this relationship the way that it was. It was while he read the letter that he admitted that he wasn't happy either. That was the only time that he said, "I've neglected you and the family."

I had never seen Karl express any emotion; I had hardly ever seen him cry, probably only once before that. Karl wouldn't get in touch with his emotions. Karl wouldn't even say, "I love you" to me. In our relationship, there was never any spontaneous embracing, holding hands, or kissing. I had seen such behaviors in others' relationships, but with my husband, I wasn't experiencing that. There just wasn't any show of affection other than sexual contact. We had sex instead of making love. My letter resulted in our talking about everything because I basically said that I couldn't stay in the marriage as it was. Karl admitted that the marriage wasn't going anywhere. We agreed that we had to let the kids know that we had decided to end our relationship. I was proud of Karl for saying to the kids that not one of us had been happy and that we had not done well with our marriage for a very long time. For once, we were like-minded in presenting to the kids the way we were.

As I reflect back on the beginning stages of our relationship, I realize that Karl never really did propose marriage to me. I was the one to ask him, "Where are we going with this relationship? Are we going to get married?" Karl would put the question back on me, "Well, what do you think?" My response was that I was ready to get married and to have a family. I feel that it was *me* who *pushed that* decision, so he went along with it, and we went ring shopping. I now think, "*Wow*, I should have just ended the relationship back then," but I guess I had high hopes that it would just keep getting better. Once I was in the marriage and I experienced the neglect, I had to stay because I didn't think that divorce was right; it wasn't the biblical thing to do.

At the same time, once the kids were out of the house and we still couldn't get on some form of closer relationship, I just couldn't see myself living the rest of my life that way! Karl secured an attorney, filed, and then I proceeded to get an attorney. It was very difficult to find support on my decision to divorce; my strongest support system was a co-worker. My closest friends were not the people I thought would be supportive because they had loyalties to both of us. There were only three to four select people in town and via social media that I felt cared, and I could trust and count on their support.

During the separation (while the divorce was in process), I attended my high school reunion. It was then that I reconnected with my childhood friend, Rob; he had been living out of state for many years. It was wonderful to catch up with Rob on where his life had taken him. Rob grew up with his hard-working mother, who divorced his alcoholic father. Rob's mother remarried, and he was raised with a stepfather whom he had a good relationship with. Other than his step-siblings, Rob's immediate family is deceased. Rob had been divorced for a couple of years; the decision to divorce was mutual after years of nonstop arguing. Rob's former wife was not supportive of a part-time business that he had out of their home, which kept him working after he got home from work and on the weekends. Rob and I exchanged stories at the reunion (I, too, updated him on my life). After that, we kept in touch through the phone, email, and social media.

Several months later when he returned to town for a visit, we dated. We fell in love. Rob proposed. We got married through my church, as he had been attending my church (even though his denomination is Baptist). We have been married for a month now. I have been divorced almost a year (eleven months.) This marriage is different because we interact with one another.

GRACE'S STORY

We're *affectionate* toward each other. We smile, we talk, gaze at each other—little things that tell you that that person loves you and feels the same way about you as you do him. This marriage is night and day compared to my marriage to Karl. Rob and I have friends outside of our marriage, but we still spend a lot of time together. I can't say enough about how different my new marriage is; my previous marriage was just a strange kind of thing.

Leaving my emotionally-abusive relationship has made a huge difference and significant impact in my life because I no longer believe what I believed before. I had it in my head that I had to stay and should not divorce. I was a firm believer that divorce was wrong, that I was to stay with him forever because I didn't want to hurt the kids. I believed that divorce was not the appropriate route to go. But separating, leaving, and actually getting the divorce has made me realize that I am a person myself and that I have a right to have my own feelings. My support system validated my feelings and beliefs, and it was—and is—the healthiest thing that I could have done! Yet, I couldn't bring myself to do it until that point.

In my former marriage, Karl was aloof and disengaged; he functioned as if he was living on his own. My emotionally-abusive marriage not only influenced my own life, but my children were affected as well. Karl was an absent parent. Karl's contact with the kids was his occasional interaction with them as opposed to outward affection. I was always the involved parent doing all of the driving, going to all of the ball games (even out of town). I was the one planning all of the birthday parties and activities. Karl wasn't involved; he was an outsider to all of it.

My children knew that, and *saw that*, on some level. As a result, my kids are all very close to me. They try to maintain equal time with their dad, but they have never been emotionally attached to him. When Karl greets his children, it's almost as if he's greeting someone that he's not close to, as if it's someone that he hasn't lived with. If the kids initiate a hug, he'll hug them back, but it's altogether different the way that he acts around them as a parent.

My abusive relationship was distant and silent. My marriage and life was very lonely. My life now is full of love, and I am content. I feel needed in my new marriage. Rob is interested in me; he converses with me; he's loving and affectionate. Rob is honest; he is *real*; he's authentic with me, and that's important. If I had to do it all over again, I would have taken more time to think through whether Karl was the one to marry. However, it's very hard to quantify that marriage because if it wasn't for that, I would not have my children.

It's important to note that if a woman is in an abusive relationship, she should get the support and therapy that she needs in order to break her cycle of abuse. It's vital that she sees herself as a person of worth and begins to believe in herself. In the short time that I have been divorced, I feel like I have been more motivated, fulfilled, and *alive* than I have been in a long, long time! I changed, and my life changed when I decided that I deserved to have happiness in my life. God's love was a factor in my changed life; *He* wants for me to be fulfilled—just as much as I want a fulfilling life. I was terribly unhappy for so many years. God wants more than anything for me to be happy; He wants all of His children to remain happy.

PART III

EMBRACING PEACE

Surrendering Your Victimization
IF A VICTIM COMES to a place of surrendering her victimization, she must arm herself with indefatigable resolve to leave her victim role for good. This is when she has decided that she has had more than enough of that dark, chaotic life—it is then and only then that she feverishly pursues the life of *peace*. The life of an *Overcomer*, as has already been reviewed, offers the victim an opportunity to exchange her living in painful distress for a safe, peaceable lifestyle. The peace of Christ is not a random act of God or an incidental occurrence but the ongoing result of living an *Overcomer* lifestyle. The transformation from living the life of a victim and becoming an *Overcomer* can bring on the experience of tranquility. As an *Overcomer*, you will be enveloped in His peace. Part of the transformation which brings peace (in addition to her spiritual peace) is her new expectation as an *Overcomer*.

Peace of mind is there because she has discovered hope and has found a resolution to her abuse trauma. She has learned the art of having the freedom to disagree with anything that's against her *Overcomer* principles without becoming disagreeable; she no longer has to over-compromise her position and apologize for it! This transformation means that she will now live on peaceful, victorious ground. However, consistent, long-lasting peace will always require assistance from the Spiritual realm. Peace is available to the victim wanting to overcome her abuse. Our God is a merciful God; it is through His mercy that He provides us with peace. All one has to do is ask for peace as it is promised in God's Word Ask for His mercy and peace—it's just a prayer away. To know that Christ's peace can live in your heart is one of the greatest pieces of all knowledge!

According to the translation of the Hebrew word *mercy*, the definition means that we are asking for God's *favor* and *grace*. When a victim asks for God's mercy in providing peace in her life, she is truly asking for His favor—which He gladly gives when she calls out to Him. Definitions of *favor* include: "to support; advocate, to make easier; help" and "to receive assistance, a special advantage or preferential treatment." Once a victim seeks and receives God's mercy and accepts His favor of her, she is able to comprehend the measure of His love. Experiencing the vastness of God's mercy (favor) and grace is an effective remedy that brings on that strength and expanse of His love and peace that is beyond human knowledge.

> "That He would grant you, according to the riches of His glory, to be strengthened with might through His Spirit in the inner man, that Christ may dwell in your hearts through faith; that you, being rooted and grounded in love, may be able to comprehend with all the saints what *is* the width and length and depth and height—to know the love of Christ which passes knowledge; that

EMBRACING PEACE

you may be filled with all the fullness of God" (Ephesians 3:16-19).

May God grant you strength with His might; He does love you immeasurably and unconditionally. The Bible speaks of David knowing the truth about God's unlimited mercy, grace, love, and the strength that only He could provide. First Samuel 30:6b says that David strengthened himself in the Lord His God. You can find motivational *Overcomer* encouraging strength in those truths, like David did. Obtaining His mercy and grace develops the knowledge of God's limitless width, length, and depth of His love, which then serves to develop His gift of peace.

The reason a victim or *Overcomer* is unable to obtain *peace* is primarily because there may be a lack of knowledge and understanding as to what inner peace is. Inner peace—when a person has reached mental and spiritual peace—is a state of being because there's enough knowledge and comprehension about the person's circumstances to keep them strong and courageous in the midst of severe stress. In some cases, peace can't be reached because there's an uncertainty as to these questions: From *Whom* is peace obtained? *Who* is peace for? And *what* is the function and purpose of peace? Peace is obtained from the Holy Spirit—God. Peace is for all human beings who ask for and pursue it. Our mind and body need peace for optimum levels of operation. The basic feelings of relaxation, contentment, and inner peacefulness fulfill a purpose by developing healthy brain processing and physical functioning. The function of peace is extensive and is not to be left intact within the person. Through inner peace, a person can expand their peace into their family system, their community, and society as a whole.

Are you ready to ask your Heavenly Father for His love and peace that surpasses all understanding? A tidal wave of His love and peace is in front of you; you can either wear your garment of suffering or His garment of love and peace. The suffering endured when deciding to leave the victim role is not peaceful unless you request and work toward inner peace. Repairing your abusive lifestyle and exchanging it for an *Overcomer* life will lead to peace. You as an *Overcomer* must cultivate peace. Plow, till, and water your garden of peace; then plant the seeds of peace, and you will harvest the fruit of peace. Are you interested in growing the fruit of peace in your life? Then...just ask for it. That is the only catch—although God's favor is always working throughout our lives, it works better if you ask for His peace favor. Expect it from Him, lest you remain in an anxious state of mind: "Be anxious for nothing, but in everything by prayer and supplication, with thanksgiving, let your requests be made known to God; and the peace of God, which surpasses all understanding, will guard your hearts and minds through Christ Jesus" (Philippians 4:6-7). Open your hand, dear one. Grasp and receive the free gift of an *Overcomer* life of peace, which Christ is generously offering to you today.

    In Mark chapter four, Jesus tells the parable of the sower (farmer). The farmer is actually God, distributing His Word like the seeds that a farmer sows. God is sowing His Word year-round. His Word is the gospel. It is sown all over the world through the Bible, sermons, literature, and whoever plants His seed (Word). It can be tilled in the soil of one's heart. Like with a farmer's soil, His seed (Word) can land on fruitful or unfruitful ground. It has the power to germinate seedlings of forgiveness, love, faith, hope, joy, and to bring about a bountiful harvest of peace in someone's spirit. The farmer has to have hope that the seeds he plants will sprout into seedlings, which will mature into a full harvest. Keeping your hope alive and your mind at rest is a direct result of God's favor and His gift of a full harvest of peace upon you. Thank you for allowing me the privilege of tilling the

EMBRACING PEACE

precious ground soil of your heart, for just a little bit. Now, are you ready to sow His peace?

If you are afraid that you will never be able to receive His favor or restore the peace you had prior to your abuse, surrender your fear and surrender your victim role; those two go hand-in-hand. Fear will cripple you and keep you from receiving favor and from restoring your peace of mind. Fear, amongst other powerful emotions, can override your intellectual thinking and produce irrational thinking and behavior. Declare, "Whenever I am afraid, I will trust in You" (Psalm 56:3). With God's love for you, and with your love for Him in return, there is no room for fear. Trust in His love to cast out your fear. "There is no fear in love; but perfect love casts out fear, because fear involves torment. But he who fears has not been made perfect in love" (1 John 4:18). "Perfect" means wholesome and complete. It does not lack anything; it is sufficient in itself. Do not allow fear to destroy your inclination to pursue a life free from your abuse. The verse says that fear involves torment. Once you seek God, fear will no longer reign supreme in your life—God's perfect love will take over fear's (torment's) place.

In Mark 4:37-39, the disciples were in a boat when a windstorm arose. The waves beat into their boat, which began to fill with water, and they panicked with fear. But Jesus rebuked the wind and said to the sea, "Peace, be still!" and the wind ceased, and there was a great calm. Do you not believe that if Jesus has the kind of power to make the wind and the waves obey Him that He can rebuke your abuse and create a calm and peace for you, just as He did for His disciples? Rebuke your abuse right now and ask Him to calm your storm and grant you peace!

Yes, releasing your fear requires a step of love and faith in God. Faith in and love for God and fear cannot cohabit in the same realm. If love and faith are predominant, there will be no room for fear; but if fear is the dominant trait, then love and faith dissolve and disappear from your livelihood. For a victim, fear can become a pattern and incapacitate her. A victim is handpicked by her Savior and handicapped in fear by the devil. It takes a radical change in love and faith habits to free up a victim from fear. A renewed, dominant love for God and a faith-based thought pattern has to become the conviction that you can do *all* things through Christ Who strengthens you (Philippians 4:13). Whether we feel God's presence or not, He is still at work in our lives. His presence through the Holy Spirit will make you strong. Trust that you can do *all* things as He says you can, and trust that He will strengthen you as He says He will! Then your fear will be the one to dissolve, and the power of your love and faith in God becomes the death-knell of your fear.

When Jesus knelt down in agony at the Garden of Gethsemane, He knew that His Heavenly Father had a plan involving Him and His crucifixion at the cross. He knew that it was for the greater good of mankind, yet He prayed to the Father to take His current suffering and the pain He knew He was about to experience on the cross away. However, in the same breath of that prayer, He surrendered for the greater good of mankind by saying to the Father, "Nevertheless, not My will, but Yours be done." Immediately after Jesus' prayer, the Bible says, "Then an angel appeared to Him from heaven, strengthening Him" (Luke 22:42-43). He can do the same for you. He will send someone or something your way when you pray and cry out in your anguish and pain—as Jesus did. You will be blessed when you surrender your victimization for *your* greater good and that of others.

Receive His Peace
Jesus Christ is the ultimate Prince of *Peace* to every human, especially to the victim who has never known or forgotten that she is royalty, the daughter of a divine King—a princess. Your Heavenly Father is the supreme God of the Universe! He is your Mes-

EMBRACING PEACE

siah that came to Earth to be your King. You have access to the One and only Highest King of the world. God's Word tells you that you are an heir—an heir of God and a co-heir with Christ. Why not accept His peace that you have inherited as a daughter in His Kingdom? "For unto us a Child is born, Unto us a Son is given; And the government will be upon His shoulder. And His name will be called Wonderful, Counselor, Mighty God, Everlasting Father, Prince of Peace" (Isaiah 9:6). He's your Prince of Peace and King, and He deserves your acclamation! Have you ever met Him? He is willing and ready to give you a well of grace and peace. Daughter of the Highest King His well of Peace is yours!

Love and the restoration of peace came upon the Samaritan woman when she met Christ at the well (John 4). Jesus showed the Samaritan woman grace, love, and compassion in spite of the downhill pattern of self-destructive living that she was undergoing. A victim can be her own worst enemy by destroying her life as the Samaritan woman was on her way to doing. Only a victim can *allow it* to be that way—Jesus won't. Christ Jesus' eyesight wants to restore your sight. He offers you spiritual insight and grit, which provides His peace, as opposed to being blind to the components of a state of peace. Christ embodies the substance of peace; peace is at the center of His being, and He wants to offer it to you. He is peace-centric. Jesus Christ is offering you a merger with Him. Merging with Christ means forgiveness (forgiveness of self, forgiveness from Him, forgiveness of others). Forgiveness is the gateway into peace and unity with Christ and others. Once the merger takes place, a way to peace is opened up.

God's love is everlasting. His Presence is in the room you're in right now. The gaze in His eyes for you is one of unbounded love. The Bible describes God's love as one of great measure, a love that's as far as the heavens are above the Earth! God's love does not encompass the scope of this book. He loves and cares about *you*; His caring over you is ineffable. "Therefore humble yourselves under the mighty hand of God, that He may exalt you in due time, casting all your care upon Him, for He cares for you" (1 Peter 5:6-7). Many victims are afraid of trusting God fully for fear that He can't be trusted because the abuser and many others have betrayed her and have become her enemy. Christ is not your enemy, no matter what your life has been like. "What then shall we say to these things? If God *is* for us, who *can be* against us?" (Romans 8:31). Christ is with the victim and is for the victim, even during those extremely painful times when His presence and favor appear absent. Christ will stop at nothing to restore you from your victimization to an *Overcomer* life. He came to live on Earth so that you would *receive His peace*. He yearns for your restoration. He desires nothing more than for you to have peace in your life. He is for you—He is on your side. That is just the way He is—because He is the Prince of Peace!

Peace is a matter of trusting God—the maker of peace. So, it's all about trust. What is trust, anyway? Some synonyms for the word "trust" are confidence, faith, and belief. Synonyms for "confidence" are secure, assured, and safe. Trusting God for providing peace means having faith and a belief in His power to restore your peace. It means finding your security in Him (even when you're hurting and He's not visible) and resting assured that you are safe with Him. He alone is powerful enough to quell your battlefield of abuse! An inability to have peace is really a lack of faith (trust), which interferes in the process of obtaining lasting peace. Believe and trust in God in equal faith. Believing in God and acknowledging His existence and presence in our Spirit is only a partial portion of faith in Him. To trust God—that He will provide for our deepest needs—is the remaining portion to doubtless faith. The word "bittachon" translated from Hebrew is "trust," which means to lean on, feel safe, or to be confident.

Trust requires leaning on God confidently in order to feel safe in all circumstances.

Undeniable trust is part of the foundation of faith, which can only be an act of a person's heart and will. When we trust God, we willingly and actively decide in our hearts that He will provide for us, and thus we place our lives in His care. Trusting God's faithfulness in Who He is and in the knowledge that He's going to do what He says He's going to do for you will dispel your fearfulness. Remember that He has commanded *us* to be faithful as well; He has commanded us to be faithful, *not* fearful. Fear, as we have learned, is not from God—never yield or surrender to fear. Fear reduces your ability to think clearly, inviting overwhelming, foggy thinking to take over. Plant the seed of faith, and trust will evolve...followed by peace. Not having peace is a serious problem to have, but an even more serious problem is not trusting Him and not believing in Him. To place full confidence in only oneself alone and to leave God out while standing apart from Him is lethal! Listen to Jesus' Words in John 15:5a: "I am the vine, you *are* the branches. He who abides in Me, and I in him, bears much fruit."

Sow your belief in Him and be a part of His vine. Not believing in Him means losing your opportunity to be His heir by not allowing Him to live within you and by not being one with Him; it means not being a part of the Father, Son, and the Holy Spirit Who brings peace. It's easy for *anyone* (not just a victim) to lack trust and not believe in the only One that can give the gift and fruit of peace. We live in a deceived culture that lives chronically in the belief system of the self only. Instead of inheriting God's everlasting peace, they inherit the world's tribulations and the epidemic of stress. He promises in His Word (the Bible) that if you believe in Him and accept Him in the midst of your circumstances, He *will* deliver peace. Peace is not all about the absence of conflict; peace is sensing and knowing the presence of God.

A steady calmness is only found in His presence, for He is the Lord of peace.

God did not promise to deliver us from the trials of daily living. He never promised that we would not be exposed to stressful human experiences. But, He does promise to be present and available for us during suffering and to encourage us and strengthen us as we pass through those painful times (that promise in itself injects peace). His peace is not about removing conflict in our relationships. The peace Christ offers is a greater peace: the kind of peace that when life takes its toll on our relationships, it will remain in our spirit to retain joy, inner strength, heal our brokenness, and promote well-being in us and others (even when others choose conflict). God is an all-knowing and all-powerful God. His Word is clear and is worthy of trust. He knows when we have given our life over to Him; He knows our heart (the state of our faith and our belief in Him). Once we have committed our life to Him, we are accountable to Him for our faith—for receiving His peace and spreading His peace, amongst other things. "Now the fruit of righteousness is sown in peace by those who make peace" (James 3:18). We are called to be peacemakers as Christ, our peace-loving leader, is. How are you able to sustain peace in an abusive relationship? How are you modeling the fruit of peace to your children and passing it on to your children's children? With God ministering to your Spirit, Mind, and Body, how can you *not* have peace? Plant the seed of belief, trust in Him, and voila, receive His peace! He freely offers His peace—receive it now.

A Personal Relationship with God Provides Peace

The Bible says that, "The fool has said in his heart, 'There is no God.'" (Psalm 14:1). But this applies to neither a victim nor an *Overcomer*. Do you believe He is alive and right there with you throughout your abuse and will be with you forever after? Something to think about when contemplating whether to believe in God, whether to accept Christ in your heart, and whether to have a personal relationship with God is this: One's identity, confidence, and security are directly connected to one's perception of God. A victim of abuse may potentially have a false perception of who God is because of her human tendency to project onto Him the abusive characteristics of the abuser or others that she has looked up to that may have deeply hurt her. She may believe that God doesn't exist because she asks where He was when she was being hurt. Or, if she believes He's real, she may think that He will also abandon her and mistreat her as others have, that He will be just like the past harmful relationships she has experienced.

Many victims feel that God will punish them because they have done things, or failed to do things, out of survival. This, of course, is an erroneous perception of God, which only leads to the victim staying away from God when she needs Him the most. This perception is completely opposite of who God is—the Father of mercies and God of all comfort (2 Corinthians 1:3). A victim's relationship with God is never about what she has done or failed to do. It's not about obeying and being a good Christian; it is all about Who God is and who you can become through God. Therefore, if a victim is to develop faith and begin a trustful relationship with God, her perception of God must be derived from God's Word—the Bible.

God loves you incessantly, unlike with the abuser ("he loves me, he loves me not"). God's love is an unending love. He awaits you to turn to Him as a victim. He beckons you to respond to His loving invitation to come to Him. When you seek Him, He will greet you with His open Arms. He will embrace you and sweetly love on you as He gently comforts and sustains you. He loves you! He loves you! He loves you! His Name is Love. Love is the core characteristic of God. He loves you with a love that exceeds all other loves. His unfathomable love for you is a pure, forgiving, cleansing love that is trustworthy. His hope is that you will be awash with the endlessness of His love. God's proclamations of His unceasing love for you are imprinted throughout the entire Bible; it is a love story which He wrote about *you*. This is the only love story that does not have a "the end" at the conclusion of the book—it is symbolic of His never-ending love for you. In His story about you (His Word), He uses the terms "unfailing love" thirty-two times to describe the love He offers you. All of Christ's acts of love are on your behalf. When He created you, He created you in love; when He speaks to you in His small, still voice, He speaks to you in love; when He guides you, He guides you in love; when He chooses for you, He chooses in love; when He disciplines you, He uses justice in love; when He overrides in His authority, He uses supremacy in His love. Love is the foundation of His character. Christ's unrequited love has no boundaries.

The love He promises you is unchanging; there is no equal. No one, apart from the Father, Son, and Holy Spirit, will ever love you more or be powerfully greater. Because of God, Christ came down from heaven for *you*—to express His love for *you*. He came to be the human expression of our Heavenly Father. If you look closely at the goodness in you and others, His attributes are visible within you and others through the Holy Spirit's power. When you decide to have faith and trust in Him, the love and security He offers is eternal. He now becomes your constant companion through the Holy Spirit. His presence will never fail to calm you and encourage you with His mercy, peace, and hope. Because of the all-encompassing aspect of His character, you will find rest and never be left comfortless. "But from there you will seek the LORD your God, and you will find *Him* if you seek Him with all your heart and with all your soul. "(for the LORD your God *is* a merciful God), He will not forsake you" (Deuteronomy 4:29, 31a). He will not forsake you because you are important to God; He longs to be a part of your journey in the life He has given you. At the same time, He sees you as the unique one whom He created. God sees you as an individual whom He loves, and He does not want harm to come your way because above all the people on the face of the Earth, you are His special treasure (Deuteronomy 7:6)!

He is your conduit to obtain love and peace. It is a love and peace that has the power to banish your anxieties, comfort you in your affliction, and enable you to cope with the trauma of abuse in the strength of your Savior. It's a comfort that helps you see hopefulness even through your tears. Won't you receive His inexpressible comfort and peace? Christ offers you His comfort through His Spirit so that you can see hope through the glaziness of your tears. If you have already accepted His comfort which He freely gives you, thank Him for it. Both the Holy Spirit and His peace are only effective when we accept and receive them. Once you receive the Holy Spirit, He will be alive and powerful within you—He will not allow you to perish in your affliction. "He shall cover you with His feathers, And under His wings you shall take refuge" (Psalm 91:4); this means that you can take comfort in, feel safe, and receive his peace under His ceaseless love and the shelter of His everlasting Arms! Are you willing to accept His gift of salvation and rest in His peace today? "I will give you rest" (Matthew 11:28c).

Surrendering your life to God is like receiving a spiritual bone marrow transplant, as it indicates in Hebrews 4:12-13: "For the word of God *is* living and powerful, and sharper than any two-edged sword, piercing even to the division of soul and spirit, and of joints and marrow, and is a discerner of the thoughts and intents of the heart. And there is no creature hidden from His sight, but all things *are* naked and open to the eyes of Him to whom we *must give* account." It's also similar to a spiritual heart transplant; God is transplanted into your heart via the Holy Spirit now living within you. Once His Word pierces your heart and you develop a relationship with Him, He becomes a part of you and you become a part of Him. He knows your thoughts and intentions, and He lets you know His intentions as well.

As has been previously mentioned, God is an intentional, relational God. He wants to impress upon you His way of thinking and being. But He can't do that if we don't have a personal relationship with Him. We may get confused and caught off-guard by the enemy's schemes to separate us from Him, but *nothing* is a surprise to Him. He is a God of peace and order, not of confusion. First Corinthians 14:33 states, "For God is not *the author* of confusion but of peace." If He has called upon you to pay attention to your life and where it is heading or not heading during your despair, He has tagged you during your deepest brokenness. He doesn't tag people who have nothing needing radical change in their lives, so consider yourself as tagged! As you work on intentionally changing your brain to a higher level of thinking, do your best not to become so academically inclined that you miss the sentimental truth. He loves you, and you are made in His Image. To live in peace is Christ—Christ *is* peace. There's a free-will choice between the Prince of Peace...or...the prince of darkness. Won't you say to Him today, "I choose You!" Don't wait until tomorrow, tomorrow can begin today! Revel in His hope and luxuriate in His relational peace now. The One Who created you knows about your dark world of abuse. He can recreate you and your world.

Sometimes abuse takes a toll on a victim's optics, and all she sees is darkness. Christ can take those dreadful dark days of your abusive life and replace them with His peace through the measureless power of His Spirit within you. Once an *Overcomer*, you'll know that while in His light you can trust Christ on dark days. Together, you and He can work intentionally to overcome your abuse. He sees and hears your daily plight, and His compassion and mercy are there waiting for your trust in Him. "*Through* the LORD's mercies we are not consumed, Because His compassions fail not. *They are* new every morning; Great *is* Your faithfulness" (Lamentations 3:22-23). When He has tagged you, He extends His Hand out to you. Confess your belief in Him and take His Hand, for if you do, you will live to see the intentional, gracious work of His Hand in your life. He offers you His peace, not just during the dark nights and days, but for the rest of your days.

God has no quotas that He has to fill. He will never meet quotas on peace because it is never too late for one more abused life to seek His peace. He is not holding off on giving you the peace that you are seeking; you're the only one that can hold things up. Peace can bring joy back into your life. You hold off on receiving His peace by being too fearful to entrust your life into His care. He promises that yesterday's victim can become tomorrow's *Overcomer,* but you need to decide today. You have been personally chosen and invited by God; He has offered you the peace of Christ. You are called to peace. Today is the day that you can take all of those tears which you have shed and sow them into the Kingdom of God so that you can reap your harvest of peace and joy! Won't you accept His peace today? "Those who sow in tears Shall reap in joy" (Psalm 126:5). Or...will you be like some people that spend their lifetime absorbing what they can from God's Word but remaining in captivity? What do I mean by this? I'm referring to those folks that have heard the good news of God's *agape* love and innumerable messages about the road to freedom and peace, studied God's Word, shed tears of agony, and even highlighted His promises, yet choose to remain consumed by suffering.

I'm talking about all the folks who have sought counsel, discovered that God's Word is the Truth, and received the revelation that Christ's love is so unconditional that He forgives our past sinful nature; *yet,* with all of His grace, they still condemn themselves and choose to remain in bondage. These folks think that they have accepted God's Word just because they have strong feelings about it. But you see, this is not enough to experience God's peace; one can receive immediate satisfaction by reading God's Word each time they open the Bible and still remain captive. Folks like these apply the biblical truths they read, such as in legalistic religion, without actually applying it to the daily underpinnings of their bondage. To have a personal relationship with Him and obtain peace, you must plow, till, plant, and water God's Word in your life daily! You must never disenroll as a student in the divine University of Overcoming—if you do—you will stop growing. It does serve you better to become a byproduct of His living water and cultivation. Taking good care of His seeds of love, grace, compassion, strength, and hope which He plants within you, will grow an overcomer garden of peace!

Most of us are familiar with the Apostle Paul; if you are not, I encourage you to read Paul's testimony in the Bible (See the books of Romans, First and Second Corinthians, and Philippians). Victims and *Overcomers* both can relate to Paul's conversion, longsuffering, and inspirational transformation of his life. I ask you the following not to cause any grain of condemnation or discomfort but to reassure you of an open-door policy with the Lord. Have you ever experienced a Paul-like moment? If you have ever lost a sense of God's presence and have regained it through faith and frequent contact with Him, you know that *nothing in the world* is worth losing God's grace and favor! Has He already made His presence known to you? Have you already entered His door of invitation, acquired a Paul-like faith, and seen Christ reveal Himself to you?

> "Behold, I stand at the door and knock. If anyone hears My voice and opens the door, I will come in to him and dine with him, and he with Me" (Revelation 3:20).

On another note, perhaps you *cannot* relate to a Paul-like moment on any level (being lost, condemning, condemned, longsuffering, and transformation). You may be saying to yourself, "But I'm a good person. I'm hard-working, honest, kind, generous, and optimistic. I stay away from bad, do good things, and never bad-mouth God." It's important to do a lot of good in life, and Paul lived that way too for a while. Being an impeccable Pharisee was Paul's measure of what it meant to be righteous with God. According to Paul's assessment before He came to Christ, he was in good standing with God; it didn't occur to him that he was being outrightly defiant in his disobedience to God when he was indifferent toward Christ. Once Paul accepted Christ as his Savior, he was able to look back on his false, carnal confidence and called it a confidence in the flesh.

Paul, like all of us, was a sinner on top of all of the good things that comprised him. Once he realized his sinful condition and experienced the conviction and condemnation that being aware of one's own sins brings, he was relieved that there was a place for grace, forgiveness, and a plan of salvation as a remedy for sin. Paul learned that he couldn't just ignore his sin, and he began to understand that no matter how much good he did, it wouldn't solve the problem of sin. Paul became passionate about discovering the plan of salvation as a solution to not having to condemn himself or being condemned in eternal damnation. Paul was now able to discern that without Christ's forgiveness of his sin, he and others like himself were lost. They were separated from God as he was—they, like him, did not have a personal relationship with God.

Paul's epiphany (that all people need no longer condemn themselves or others but instead read, listen, believe and become obedient to God's Word to receive Christ's forgiveness and relationship) was a transformation that led him to share the good news. Even though we are sinners, Christ's followers are *not* condemned. He instead invites us into fellowship with Him in spite of our sin; we don't have to remain separated from Christ because of our sin. Paul spells out the plan of salvation very simply and clearly through his testimony and ministry to others: Jesus Christ died, but even after we sinned against Him, He proved His love for us and told us that we were *not* condemned for that sin. He forgave us for that past sin and remains today as an advocate for any of our sins once we invite Him into our life. "My little children, these things I write to you, so that you may not sin. And if anyone sins, we have an Advocate with the Father, Jesus Christ the righteous" (1 John 2:1).

God's Word is explicit; once we become aware of our sinful nature, there's only one way out of self-condemnation—through the plan of salvation. There's only one problem that remains to be solved once sin is brought to one's awareness, and that's the basic requirement of a trusting relationship (which we have already discussed). It takes the participation of more than one person to have a bonded relationship! In order to receive the plan of salvation, a person has to accept and commit to a personal relationship with Jesus Christ. Christ will not be ringing your doorbell today to ask you if you want to be forgiven. Forgiveness, making amends with God, and the removal of self-condemnation will not happen automatically once you learn about the plan of salvation. He will remain standing there at your door, waiting for you to ask for His forgiveness. You must, like Paul, act upon your new spiritual knowledge and respond with faith and obedience to the plan. He won't twist your arm and ask for your apologies. You have to personally respond by accepting His invitation to come into your life and asking for His forgiveness. You have to let Him in the door, and once forgiven, you can begin your new life walking daily in His presence.

God's peace will only come to us if we yield to Him; that's what Paul ultimately did to receive God's peace. God's peace can only infiltrate us through our personal relationship with Him. Once we receive His peace, we are able to discern, like Paul, what *is* and what is *not* of God. You will know and recognize God's peace as opposed to the world's (or satan's) because God's peace is always separated by that which is pure and true and beams with light, not darkness. Perhaps, you're still back there in the dark, wallowing in the senseless hardships that you've had to endure. Ultimately, staying in the past was not an option for Paul. It's truly not an option for any of us unless we choose to dwell on the past. Through grace, peace leads a victim out of a past wrongful lifestyle. Peace and abuse do not go hand-in-hand; a healthy marriage is not possible without peace, and we're unable to have a relationship with God without peace between God and ourselves (Ephesians 2:14-18). An *Overcomer* discovers that the only lasting solution to her victimization comes from Christ. She realizes that He's the only One Who can give her abiding peace. Peace is the hallmark of an *Overcomer*. God has called you to peace (1 Corinthians 7:15)!

God Advocates for Your Peace
If God is offering to advocate for you, to crush satan, the maker of warfare, and give you peace, why would you *not* accept His invitation? "And the God of peace will crush satan under your feet shortly" (Romans 16:20). I'm not by any means undermining your pain, for I know it hurts even to recollect what you have been through, especially if you're still searching for some answers for why you've lived through this abuse trauma. I respect your desire for explanations and answers from God, and some

day you may have some answers from Him. In the meantime, stay with me here; some meanings and purposes for your life will become more comprehensible as this book reaches closure. Do you need *more* good news? All *Overcomers* do! Can you handle some more inspirational reading? I'm going to share some thoughts about how others in the Bible handled their joys and their sorrows.

The Bible has numerous examples of the difference between those that acknowledge God in how they live their lives compared to those who live their lives without God's guidance. Amongst the sixty-six books in the Bible, the middle book of Psalms radiates David's and other believers' reflections on being blessed by knowing God. In these people's lives, there are peak periods of joy along with manifestations of pain and suffering alike. Nevertheless, it becomes quite clear in the Psalms that believing in God is not quite sufficient to receive the blessings of peace in their lives. The Psalms compare people that ignore or deliberately despise God with those that receive the joy of having God in their life; the latter revere God. God created all of us to be *Overcomers*, but in order for us to be successful in overcoming all that this life brings our way, we have to submit to His Godhead or we could fail to live a righteous life in Him. He did not create us to be failures at doing life, but the reality is that without Him, we can fail in life by default.

The Psalms reveal a people that search for God with all of their heart and, therefore, discover and follow His ways. When the psalmists cried out and submitted to God, God showed up and advocated for them! It is a matter of choosing in our life whom we will submit to and what we will embrace. The Bible teaches us to submit only to that which is of God. There is either Christ in a person or satan in them. When we submit to Christ in a person (His Image), we're submitting to God, and we become more like His Image. If a person submits to satan in any part(s) of their life, then they resemble his likeness. We submit to whatever we serve, and it becomes our god. We are not to make a god out of others. Won't you submit to *God* and embrace *His peace*?

The Bible makes it evident that His ways are righteous, and following His ways (no matter how trying the circumstances) will *always* be not, only the right way, but also the path to your everlasting peace. It's obvious in the Psalms that those who do not have a place for God in their lives carry the burden of being their own god, which does not deliver peace in their souls. Quite the contrary, being their own god brings on misery and grows into a malignancy in their souls. When a person submits to God, He knows what decisions you are to make and speaks to you about these through His Holy Spirit. As evidenced in the Psalms, the blessing of submitting to God and obedience to Him is the way to healing and restoration—the way to peace. Try as you may, you will never in your entire life be able to find a circumstance in which God's guidance isn't the best route!

Oh, the immense peace that takes over when the obstacles of abuse are removed through repentance and a changed Spirit, Mind, and Body. It's possible that you have been fearful of God or even angry at Him, but if you've ever had a curiosity about Him or even had a past relationship with Him, you know how empty that void is when you have Him at arm's length. Re-invite Christ into your heart; restore His presence in your Spirit. He promises to advocate for you to the Father. He will intercede for you (Romans 8:34). Christ is sitting at the right Hand of God right now interceding for you—He is your personal Mediator!

He is a "yes" God; He keeps *all* of His promises if you seek Him. "For all the promises of God in Him *are* Yes, and in Him Amen, to the glory of God through us" (2 Corinthians 1:20). Invite Him to abide within you, and He will reveal Himself to you via His Word. He will instill a supernatural awakening inside you about His presence and authority as He completes His promises to you. He can never abide in you without bringing His peace into your soul; He can never be near your presence without pouring His blessings upon you. When your abuse mars your vision and escalates your fear, turn to Christ. Overcome your abuse through the peace of His presence. Call out to Him—He is for your being and not against you. Or, listen for His calling on you today. Our response is all He has ever asked for—for us to say *yes* to Him when He calls us. Out in the heavens, the angels are waiting to sing, dance, and celebrate your restoration with Him! "Likewise, I say to you, there is joy in the presence of the angels of God over one sinner who repents" (Luke 15:10). Humble yourself and respond to His calling, and as your heart beats, whether it's a painful, desperate, or an excited beat, take His peace and own It!

The Power of Humility & His Forgiveness
We're back to humility of the soul. Before acknowledging God, we have to admit that He's supreme and that we are human in dealing with our circumstances. This is not to be confused or misunderstood with the supremacy of authoritarian domination; that would be a form of dogmatic religious legalism. This form of religious doctrine would only further oppress God's people. The God of the Bible, although supreme and in authority, *does not* oppress; He delivers His people from oppression. Furthermore, it is important to know that our God is not interested in what has led to your circumstances of oppression. Once you submit your life in humility to Him, His love and defense of you is all that matters to Him!

You have surrendered your heart and have returned to Him Who created you; that's all that He cares about. Your return to Him and your crying out to Him in need is His only concern. God's love and forgiveness is offered freely, not because we're entitled—but because of His hearing and answering of our cry with His unlimited grace. It's all about fastening your mind on Him and securing His presence in your life. If you decide that you're undeserving because some of your own decisions and poor choices have magnified your situation, then you should trust God's Word that your part in the situation only merits confessing and accepting His forgiveness and fully expecting His mercy, deliverance, and redemption. "Hope in the LORD; For with the LORD *there is* mercy, And with Him *is* abundant redemption" (Psalm 130:7).

Even if you believe in your mind that your unbelief, idolatry of things or others, or deliberate disobedience of His commands is what engulfed your oppression, He *does not* keep an active record on Earth of what led you to your oppression—the only record that's in heaven is when *you* are recorded in the Lamb's Book of Life (Philippians 4:3, Revelation 3:5, 13:8, 20:15, 21:27). You can choose to be saved and recorded in the Book of Life anywhere and anytime that you are ready to give up living in an oppressed state. If you choose to take God's direction, you will no longer feel oppressed in your circumstances because you have elected to walk in His ways—no longer oppressed, just walking in *His love*.

You can also choose to postpone receiving a personal relationship with God. God will not coerce you into a relationship with Him. He is not just a Deity that looks down from heaven and prides Himself on how many people worship Him. He is a *real God* who is sensitive to your thoughts and feelings, and He seeks your relationship with Him—not your idolatry. God is truly tuned into the frequency of your contact with Him. As you get to know Him better, you will note that the frequency of your contact with Him is the measure of your faith, and it will determine the level of peace you will experience. He can't hear your desperation for hope and peace of mind if your shattered heart does not seek Him and His precepts.

We've discussed how God's plan for your life is *not* to live in the heartache of abuse; those are satan's plans. Any plans of hurt, chaos, and hopelessness for your life are easy to identify because they are satan's plans and *au contraire* to God's. Beware of being deceived by satan that hope and peace are unattainable while you're in your hopeless state of mind (Colossians 2:8, 10). satan is not interested in your peace of mind; he is not of peace—just like your abuser is not about peace. satan is not your friend; he's your fiend! God is your friend: "No longer do I call you servants, for a servant does not know what his master is doing; but I have called you friends, for all things that I heard from My Father I have made known to you" (John 15:15). God's plan is founded and grounded in His love for you. satan has the opposite in mind for you.

I would like to take a moment to illustrate my warning to you about your enemy—the great deceiver. To bring the point home to you, I am going to write out the direct *opposite* of the following Scripture verse that demonstrates God's love for you (John 3:16-17):

> "For God so loved the world that He gave His only begotten Son, that whoever believes in Him should not perish but have everlasting life. For God did not send His Son into the world to condemn the world, but that the world through Him might be saved."

I have rewritten John 3:16-17 in reverse, *exposing satan* and how he feels about you and the world:

> "For satan so hated the world that he gave nothing, that whosoever believes in him should perish and have the everlasting nether world. For satan

sent his followers into the world to condemn the world, so that the world through him might be lost."

No matter what abuse has done to you and your loved ones, you are *loveable* and *worthy* of hope and peace in your life. Don't permit satan to tell you otherwise. Always remember that satan's goal is to deceive and disturb your peace, just like when he deceived the first woman God created in paradise. His deceptive way is as old as the garden in which he found the woman. Oh yes, satan's old garden trick! satan presents his underhanded scheme to rob you of your peace, hoping his crafty attentiveness will convince you that he has the better offer, such as he offered Eve! Don't let him steal your garden of peace. When you humble yourself and reach out to God for His help from the depths of despair (taking full responsibility for your life, the good and the sin), He *is* present. You may have been absent from God's presence and may have fallen short of His glory, but He would never be tardy or truant in your life. He's ready to appear in your life whenever you're ready to receive Him. If you put your full trust in God and His Word, He is there in your presence.

We may have failed God by not loving Him unconditionally or by not turning to Him for His help, but He never fails us because His love is unfailing! "The LORD has appeared of old to me, *saying,* 'Yes, I have loved you with an everlasting love; Therefore with lovingkindness I have drawn you'" (Jeremiah 31:3). Pray that satan will *not* outwit you. Bind satan, who reeks with prideful assurances that you don't need to ask for forgiveness or pursue peace. You can have God's peace if you overcome satan, your enemy—the author of victimization. Submitting to satan's lies keeps a victim deceived. It will only be the victim that gives satan cooperative permission to keep her captive in his schemes.

God has anointed Jesus with the Holy Spirit and the power to heal all those who are oppressed by satan (Acts 10:38).

God is on to satan. He is privy to all of his schemes, and He will heal you and protect you from his enticing snare! Cling to the Lord, not unto the great deceiver. Humble yourself unto the One Who is the *Truth* and loves you with an everlasting love. Ask the Lord to give you a higher bounty of discernment to know the truth and readily identify satan's crafted lies. God says that satan's lies about you are already defeated; Christ's love and beliefs about you are indestructible. While satan hovers over you, telling you that you're "not good enough," Christ is leaning in, gently whispering in your ear, "You are good enough. In fact, you are more than enough!" The Lord (not satan) is the love and hub of your life. Humbly give yourself unto the One Who loves you unconditionally and Whose Truth sets you free. With His love and protection, you and He are untouchable! Once you leave the victim role, you walk only in Truth, and you latch onto Christ's forgiving light. You become a threat to satan's lies and his kingdom of darkness—such as Jesus is. satan is just an impediment. Christ is Truth. A victim who walks humbly into Truth and Forgiveness walks in freedom.

God's Love Restores You
God's love rises above all abusive acts. The problem of abuse trauma is deep...but God's love is deeper! *Nothing* compares to the love Christ has to offer. No human or any other temptation by the enemy can fulfill a human's need for love. In the book of Lamentations, we read about the prophet Jeremiah and how he experiences devastating circumstances as victims do that leave him emotionally depleted. Jeremiah felt alone and without human support; his own people rejected him (see Lamentations 3:13-20). Jeremiah came to many a low point, yet, in his darkest hours, Jeremiah considered God's unfailing love as he penned:

"'The LORD *is* my portion,' says my soul, 'Therefore I hope in Him!'" (Lamentations 3:24).

We can choose to live by human love alone, but there's a danger in that choice—the danger of misplaced trust. Jeremiah equips us with God's insight about misplaced trust: "Thus says the LORD: 'Cursed *is* the man who trusts in man And makes flesh his strength, Whose heart departs from the LORD'" (Jeremiah 17:5). If you're feeling betrayed by your abuser, who was supposed to be your loving companion and your friend, and others who don't validate your abuse and who are not supportive of your disunion with an abuser, read Psalm 55. It is a Psalm that correlates with the suffering of a victim and the approach taken as an *Overcomer*. The Psalmist laments and grieves because he feels surrounded only by enemies and feels the pain even more so because one of his closest friends is the betrayer. The Psalmist resolves to remain faithful to God and to trust in Him regardless. Read it! It will both inspire you and give you an encouraging booster.

If we put our trust in God, He will not disappoint us. Humans can fail us because they are just as vulnerable as we are. Humans may vow to love us forevermore yet fail to maintain that promise, but God's love is untainted and never fails; it remains steadfast and certain. Steadfastness is the benchmark of God's love. He will never say, "I don't love you anymore." His love exceeds human love. He loved you when He created you and when you were born, and He will love you until you're at your deathbed. His love for you will never decrease; He will carry on loving you. Even when you fall into the temptation of sin, you can always return to reconcile with God. When you seek and receive God's love, it will unfold within you with all of His glory, teaching you to love yourself as He does and to love others as He loves you. Now that's a deep love which you can trust *and* can count on!

Jesus Christ has an invitation for each of us: to receive His love and redemption. We, in turn, can accept His invitation and at the same time offer our own invitation to allow Him into our lives—to change our lives. But before we invite Him in, we must come forward with an attitude of humility, conviction, and cooperation. Through confessing our disownment of Him, our sins, and our submission to Him, He can restore our purity of Spirit, Mind, and Body, our whole well-being.

If you are to experience the true significance of peace in your life, your spiritual tug-of-war with God must come to an end now. In order to submit to our Creator, we must naturally decrease our human ego. As has been examined, to have true intimacy with God, one must begin at ground zero with a humbled mindset. This is what an *Overcomer* attitude looks like. An *Overcomer* attitude is what invites Christ to restore a victim of abuse. This restoration is what empowers an *Overcomer* to regain her identity and equips her with a supernatural ability to heal the self and help other victims to heal along the way. A restored victim becomes an *Overcomer* whose warfare is now her mission field. The following Scriptures are written out for you to read and ponder over God's love and promises of peace for you:

> "As the Father loved Me, I also have loved you; abide in My love" (John 15:9).

> "For I am persuaded that neither death nor life, nor angels nor principalities nor powers, nor things present nor things to come, nor height nor depth, nor any other created thing, shall be able to separate us from the love of God which is in Christ Jesus our Lord" (Romans 8:38-39).

EMBRACING PEACE

"But God demonstrates His own love toward us, in that while we were still sinners, Christ died for us" (Romans 5:8).

"Therefore, having been justified by faith, we have peace with God through our Lord Jesus Christ" (Romans 5:1).

"For He Himself is our peace, who has made both one, and has broken down the middle wall of separation" (Ephesians 2:14).

"I will both lie down in peace, and sleep; for You alone, O Lord, make me dwell in safety" (Psalm 4:8).

"The Lord will give strength to His people; the Lord will bless His people with peace" (Psalm 29:11).

"For the mountains shall depart And the hills be removed, But My kindness shall not depart from you, Nor shall My covenant of peace be removed," Says the Lord, who has mercy on you" (Isaiah 54:10).

As you finish reading and pondering over these Scriptures (which depict the dimensions of His love and His covenant of peace), meditate on the following Scripture and put your own name in the blank while you listen for God's voice as He speaks to you through this verse:

"You will keep _____ in perfect peace, *whose* mind *is* stayed *on You,* Because _____ trusts in You" (Isaiah 26:3).

Some people in the world, as a result of ignorance, fear, or pure naivety regarding a personal relationship with God, misinterpret Christianity as a neurotic, helpless dependence on religion. God's Word—His truth—was not written to be misinterpreted or misunderstood. His Word makes it clear that a personal relationship with Him is simply a trusting relationship that is available to all. No one is a simpleton or a victim of Christ. In a relationship with God, the contrary is true—He is a God who loves us all and desires nothing less than for us to be free to overcome any form of oppressed neurotic dependence! We are not God's victims—we are His beloved children that He created. Think of the love you have for your own children; imagine a love in a divine and multiplied capacity; that's His love for you. He has no ill will for you or any hidden agendas for your mental well-being (only satan does). He desires for you to experience His peace.

Yes, God is a mysterious God in some aspects of our life, but there is a myriad of insights that God reveals and enlightens us on as we consider and contemplate His Word. When we mentor, educate, and share God and His Word with others, He guides us with His wisdom regarding our audience's capacity to receive the things of Him and His Kingdom. Those things that remain a mystery are meant to remain a mystery because they belong to God as He fulfills His purpose for each of us and His world. So, what does one say to these unanswered mysteries or questions regarding whether they will have peace or not? Don't ask, "Got Peace?" Ask, "Got God?" If you have God *daily,* you can have *peace.*

Many may answer the question, "Do you have God?" like those that have grown up in church all of their life: "Of course, I do." Growing up and listening to the gospel all of your life is not a qualifier for knowing God or His peace. Many Christians know God from early childhood, and that's exactly where they left Him. He has simply been sitting on the shelf while they continue to attend church or go about their life. God didn't create us so that we could leave Him as a past experience. Neither did He create us so that we could dust Him off someday in the future whenever we feel like it. He can't offer, express, or restore us with His love if we're not available to be restored. He created us to be in relationship with Him, which can't happen if you leave Him behind as a past experience or are waiting to deal with Him in the future.

It's unfortunate, but many Christians treat God this way and then they wonder why they don't have peace in their life. Many of these Christians received Christ as an automatic inheritance along with their last name. They didn't have to do anything to experience God; He was already a part of their family. They got used to the ritual of carrying a Bible around and attending, even serving, in church; however, the rest of the time, God just sits like décor on a shelf (regardless of their having accepted salvation). There's a divine difference when someone receives God's love with a broken spirit (convicted repentance) and accepts Him, not as a nostalgic experience in their life, but as a part of their daily, present, ongoing life, which leads to a future eternity with Him. Have you ever noticed the spiritually-divine hilarity within someone who has received Christ and His love, someone with a broken, humble spirit who lives Christ daily, compared to someone who has received Christ and His love but leaves Him and His Word on a shelf?

God's Word Renders Peace
Evangelist Dwight L. Moody said, "The Bible was given not for our information but for our transformation." I can't say this enough: God's Word was written to be consistently applied to *every* detail of one's life. God's Word was penned not only to read about Him, but also to spend time with Him. As with any close relationship, it takes time to build, and if the relationship is neglected, it will become a distant relationship and eventually deteriorate. One can have no relationship with God, a lukewarm relationship with God, or a deep, intimate relationship with Him. Once put into action, reading His Word can grow you into His Image. In addition, select someone or multiple folks who are ahead of you spiritually that can mentor you. Reading His Word is not just to receive His instructions but about your formation in Christ. Beyond folks in general and onto the victim of abuse, why do victims attend Christian individual and group therapy, seminars, worship services, and Bible studies and yet don't move on to receive His Love and His peace? Because they have not yet realized that it's not about feeling emotionally touched or moved by God's Word; it's about becoming intimate with Him and being moved into action through His Truth-filled Word.

A victim can sit during a sermon and "Amen!" the pastor under her breath when he preaches on Christ's love and peace that is available; yet, she can return home unchanged and with no plan to take any steps toward peace. "Amen" in Hebrew means "so be it." Own the meaning of *Amen*, instead of leaving God on the shelf. A victim can decide that the message was not meant for her, thinking that surely God didn't mean for her to accept His love and peace and apply it to *her* life, knowing how devastating her home life is. The victim needs to not question God's thinking and the message that she just heard—she needs to ask her own self as she returns to her bondage, "What am I thinking?!"She needs to also think about that sermon on Christ's love and peace as *Amen*—so be it with me!

Please know that my thinking is not one of judging your hurtful, difficult life; they are instead thoughts of you living to receive His peace and wanting for you to open up your eyes to reap His most precious gifts for you—the promises of His strength and His peace (Psalm 29:11). God's promises of His peace are found all over His Word. He also promises to grow you in faith, love, and joy embraced with that peace! There are many folks who get impatient with God and charge God with His unfaithfulness in fulfilling His promises, forgetting that God's message has always been that in time we reap what we sow. "And let us not grow weary while doing good, for in due season we shall reap if we do not lose heart" (Galatians 6:9). If we only read and hear about God's peace and we don't get down in action on our knees, praying and following up with steps of faith, then it's just about great theological promises of peace and not a realized reality. He is faithful in being a merciful God of grace who will listen to your plea for peace. But, praying for peace for self and others is insufficient without applying the practical action steps that will lead to peace. It is like aspiring to stay fit; it becomes difficult to achieve if self-discipline, a good nutritive regimen, and exercise are not daily actions toward that goal. Won't you take small, daily steps of faith? A little step-of-faith at a time is much when God's involved!

Consider the Parable of the Sower as it is explained by Christ in Luke 8:11-15:

> "Now the parable is this: The seed is the word of God. Those by the wayside are the ones who hear; then the devil comes and takes away the word out of their hearts, lest they should believe and be saved. But the ones on the rock *are those*

who, when they hear, receive the word with joy; and these have no root, who believe for a while and in time of temptation fall away. Now the ones *that* fell among thorns are those who, when they have heard, go out and are choked with cares, riches, and pleasures of life, and bring no fruit to maturity. But the ones *that* fell on the good ground are those who, having heard the word with a noble and good heart, keep *it* and bear fruit with patience."

If you have been hearing God's Word, even if you have not been attentive, our very intentional God has been seeking your attention. If you go beyond paying attention and decide to patiently apply (obey) His Word to your abusive circumstances, you can open up the door to capture His love and His peace. Capturing His love and being captured by His love is the only form of captivity you would ever want to experience. Prolonging closeness to His love will only prolong your abusive captivity. A friend of our family prefers to be a part-time Christian. She doesn't want to fully commit to a daily walk with God because there are still some things that she wants to be able to do that she knows wouldn't quite meet God's approval; so, she is waiting to make her full-time commitment later on. Coming from a very dark, broken, unlovable family background, this person could certainly use some divine peace in her life. However, she's going to wait to apply God's Word in her life. She will be sowing her pain and her faith later—whenever that is. How about you? Are you going to sow your faith in Him and His Word today so that you can reap His promises and harvest your first fruits of peace sooner rather than later? It is never too late to return to God if you know Him but have not been abiding in Him. You can always ask Him to abide in you and your life anew. Abide in Him. Be one with Him!

Take a moment now and read John 15:4-5. After reading it, reflect upon its meaning and personalize this Scripture. Add to the second person by filling in *your name* in the blanks:

> "Abide in Me, and I in you____. As the branch cannot bear fruit of itself, unless it abides in the vine, neither can you____, unless you____ abide in Me. I am the vine, you____ *are* the branches. He who abides in Me, and I in him, bears much fruit; for without Me you____ can do nothing."

Maybe you're still feeling uneasy or skeptical about reading God's Word; if so, do a trial read. Pray for God's Spirit to accompany you as you read. Read one book of the Bible. Read John. If after you've read it, you do not discover the existence of God and you do not experience an encounter with the nature, personality, and character of God the Father, Son, and Holy Spirit, then pray for the mystery of His existence to be revealed to you, and He will do it! This is the very reason that Jesus, our Savior, came down from heaven and ministered the gospel—so that you and I and the world would meet and greet God, get to know Him, and experience the rest of our lives with His Presence (the Light of the world). "In Him was life, and the life was the light of men. And the light shines in the darkness, and the darkness did not comprehend it" (John 1:4-5); "I am the light of the world. He who follows Me shall not walk in darkness, but have the light of life" (John 8:12).

It is God's will that we experience His light and not remain in darkness. "I have come *as* a light into the world, that whoever believes in Me should not abide in darkness" (John 12:46). Whether or not you can understand and feel His light shining into your darkness, it will remain there until you're ready to behold it. God's Word is always available to introduce you to and lead you to His light *and* to light the path ahead of you. There is no expiration date on God's Word. Whenever you pick up His Word to read, it will render peace unto you through His immortal light. "Your word *is* a lamp to my feet And a light to my path" (Psalm 119:105). Translated from the Scriptures, the lamp symbolizes the wisdom, knowledge, and guidance that the light of God's Word provides; so that we will not stumble and fall.

Accept His Peace
Peace, "Shalom"—used in the Bible as the Jewish word, which means "to be complete or whole" or "to be sound" or "to live well"—can be yours! If you cannot seem to move yourself over to a place of being productive in developing the fruit of peace, then there may be a stronghold keeping you from abiding in Him. The term "stronghold" can be also be used to identify a place of protection from attack, such as a fortress. An example can be the Lord becoming our stronghold, such as in Psalm 18:2 whereby the Lord protects us from satan. But, at this time, I'm referring to *stronghold* as a metaphor representing human reliance (a self-life) as opposed to relying on God's guidance.

These types of strongholds are the wrong attitudes that we use to defend ourselves when our self-life is questioned. This self-life is the dwelling (stronghold) of satan's oppression on a person's life. Maintaining a self-life gives satan an influential place in a person's thought-life. Basically, your negative attitude toward being open to God provides a dwelling place for satan in your life. A victim must simply get to a place of seeking God's peace because despair just waves a white flag to satan and invites a partnership with him (a stronghold). As a victim, instead of leading a self-life and telling God how *you* want your life to be constructed, let God tell you how *He* wants you to construct

EMBRACING PEACE

your life; after all, He created the blueprint. He's got the master plan!

God asks us to sow righteousness by seeking Him. He warns us not to trust just having our own way. He promises that when we seek Him, we will reap His mercy. He reminds us that we have Him to overthrow whatever problem or devastation we're facing—that we're not called to depend solely on our own perceptions, discernment, or strength, and that when on fallow ground, we should not eat the fruit of deception, satan's lies (Hosea 10:12-13). Examine yourself. Do you trust only in your own ways? Are you eating satan's fruit of lies? Seek the Lord first and trust His ways so that you may reap His righteousness in your life. If you allow the Hand of God to work in your life, and if you allow Him to divinely direct all of your life affairs in order for Him to fulfill His purpose in you, you shall experience His peace.

Some of the circumstances in your life may not change, but the circumstances in your Mind and Spirit are changed in the midst of them (as you keenly feel God's presence in every area of your life). An *Overcomer* that experiences God's peace is one who reveres Him, accommodates her life around Him, and follows His ways. A victim that has been in the captivity of abuse (prior to her release as an *Overcomer*) receives a renewed spirit. She is now captivated by His love. God takes first place in an *Overcomer*'s life. He is her way of life. The end result of such a commitment to her God is that her life now operates at an optimal healthy balance, experiencing the joy of not living a self-guided self-life but instead one of purposeful peace.

Is fear of surrendering your abuse and your life to Christ still paralyzing you? After educating yourself on the dynamics of your abuse and having been reassured that you can be delivered from fear, if you are still allowing fear to torment you, that fact becomes a stronghold for satan. Fear is a sin-habit because you are choosing fear over having faith that God can deliver you from fear of anything. Fear will continue to dominate your life even after much counsel, with little avail, because you have not yet accepted humility of the mind. We have already discussed the vital importance of humbling yourself unto the Lord if you're going to become obedient and follow His lead. Your spirit of fear must be addressed as a stronghold of fear that has to be bound and cast down such as satan is. A victim freed from satan's petrified fear becomes an *Overcomer* who releases the stronghold of destructive fear in exchange for a divine nature that expands her view of God and life.

It's not true that because you have the Holy Spirit living within you, you cannot be deceived by a stronghold (satan). That is the very reason the Holy Spirit was sent as a helper and discerner of truth because humans can easily fall into self-deception. Once satan deceives you, it is extremely difficult to recognize that you have been deceived. To obtain the humility of mind that the Bible speaks on, one must totally surrender their life to Christ; not doing so renders one vulnerable to satan ruling their heart and mind. That is the very reason it is of first importance to establish a personal relationship with God. Once we have that personal relationship established, it means we are willing to conform to God's character and to allow His power to transform us into the Image of Christ. In order to establish this relationship with God and develop into His Image, it becomes necessary to remove all of our old, unproductive ways of thinking and doing so that Christ can support the removal our strongholds as He manifests Himself in us.

There are victims whose desire to be set free from the stronghold of abuse leads to *nothing* simply because they're too afraid to take the risk of making an effort. These victims' potential to overcome their abuse is lost because they rely only on themselves and unhelpful resources. The end result is that they rob themselves of the opportunity to be set free from their stronghold and they sabotage the experience of peace in their life. No one in the history of the Bible who was called by God had the expertise and energy to undertake the challenge that was allotted to them, in their own strength. With insurmountable challenges—in our own strength—we have nothing to offer. But, through the Spirit of God we can become powerful and effective in our strength. Negligence and weakness of the self are not in God's vocabulary nor plan for you (that's satan's jargon and project). Christ has a challenge for you today. If you would surrender your stronghold of abuse to Him and pursue His guidance through prayer, He will not only lead you to what you should do, but He will also send the Holy Spirit to inspire you with the training and ability to undertake your stronghold and lead you to freedom from abuse, in His Name.

Perhaps you are able to rely on God at times, but that is not true abiding because abiding is constant, enduring, and permanent. A loophole in occasionally exalting the self above the knowledge of God gives satan a place in your mind. Strongholds are similar to when people disassociate (deflect pain by escaping into avoidance/denial/blocking or continuing to do more of the same); they build barriers around their belief system and emotions to barricade and protect themselves from experiencing additional pain. In the same way that openly dealing with disassociation is healing, so it is through divine intervention on strongholds.

A significant part of the process of healing and transformation is to identify and remove the strongholds that attack and perpetuate in the wounded spirit. Once strongholds are identified and admitted to (instead of defending or excusing our thoughts or behaviors), it is at that point that we have humbled ourselves and, in faith, trust God to change our old ways. It is only then that a person can be delivered from their stronghold(s).

What action(s) on your behalf will incur the divine blessing of peace? satan would prefer for a person to remain in captivity by a stronghold (sin-habit) because if the stronghold stays, then satan can rob the person of God's power, peace, and joy. Deal with satan once and for all when it comes to your stronghold *in the same way* that Christ dealt with satan before he went to the cross. Christ said, "he has nothing in Me" (John 14:30). Declare as Christ does that satan doesn't have any living quarters inside of you!

When satan's strongholds have been overthrown in your mind (even if you occasionally miss a step), Christ will be there to hold your right hand as you victoriously overcome your abuse and not only experience deliverance, but also gain the ability to walk others through their deliverance. There is deliverance from dark, destructive strongholds. The Lord promises! "Shall the prey be taken from the mighty, Or the captives of the righteous be delivered? But thus says the LORD: 'Even the captives of the mighty shall be taken away, And the prey of the terrible be delivered; For I will contend with him who contends with you, And I will save your children'" (Isaiah 49:24-25). He not only promises to contend with your abuser, and to set you free from captivity, but He also reassures you of His eternal love and kindness toward you; it's not just a promise—it is a covenant. "'For the mountains shall depart And the hills be removed, But My kindness shall not depart from you, Nor shall My covenant of peace be removed,' Says the LORD, who has mercy on you" (Isaiah 54:10).

Christ demonstrated to us through His kindness toward all (even sinners) what love is; love is kind. Genuine love is expressed only when it is accompanied by kindness amongst the other fruit of the Spirit. As we have discussed, one of the major strongholds that a victim has to surrender in order to receive God's loving peace is fear. God's Word includes at least 365 vers-

EMBRACING PEACE

es that contain the *do-not-be afraid* admonition. That is a daily reminder that He wants to ratify that message in your Spirit, emphatically reveal it in your Mind, and proclaim it to your Body: "Do not fear." Fear can overtake you as a paralytic stronghold. Christ does not turn a blind eye to fear. Instead, He intervenes on our blurred vision. He repeatedly warns us not to be overcome by fear—instead, He compels us to overcome fear! Christ is willing and able to turn your fear into a blessing of peace. He is your Fearless Leader. How calming is that?!

The constancy of God's peace can be had in the midst of enormous fear. There is an ample supply of peace in Christ. He alone can guarantee you His redemptive peace of mind. Go to Him; receive all of His love, mercy, wisdom, power, comfort, and peace supplied. Ask not or ask for little, and you will receive such. Ask for much peace and you will receive such as you ask. His peace like His love, mercy, comfort, wisdom, and power are inexhaustible! They are all wrapped up ready to gift you—all stored up—in Christ. If you ask, Christ Himself will grant you peace!

Though satan assaults you with the torment of fear, you can rest in the fact that Christ has offered His peace and should you accept it, this can be deposited into your account of His promises—a place where you can make unlimited withdrawals and each time receive a sense of being still in His quiet peace. It takes Christ's interventions—until all the abuse storms that are as lightning puncturing and burning your soul—are calmed into His peaceful tranquility.

God has extended an invitation to you to accept and receive His peace. If you're serious about your quest for personal peace, rest assured that you need not grieve your sorrows anymore; He has already done that for you. Christ took our sinful nature and all of our sorrows on Himself so that He could forgive us, and we could have peace with His Father—God. That peace can live in each of our hearts if we choose the freedom peace brings. The only true freedom a human can experience is the peace of God in their heart. There is no peace to be found out in the world. God did create the world, but the world to Him is but a small parenthesis in heaven (eternity). Heaven is eternally bigger than Earth. In the scope of life and the eternal plan He has for you, the abusive life you have been living is a parenthesis as well in comparison to the proposed *Overcomer* life He has planned for you! Abide in Him and His Word.

The seed of the fruit of peace is the Word of God. He *does* produce the fruit of the Spirit, one of them being peace; He *removes* strongholds and *does* restore peace! Whatever your sorrows, none of them are too unbearable for God. Won't you relinquish and give Him your sorrows? "Surely He has borne our griefs And carried our sorrows; But He was wounded for our transgressions, He was bruised for our iniquities; The chastisement for our peace was upon Him, And by His stripes we are healed" (Isaiah 53:4-5). God's blessings come in many ways and sometimes at bewildering times, but His peace can be obtained right now—if you only *ask for it*. To have an abundant life, you must obtain the absolute embodiment of peace that only He can give. Abuse offers dispeace; overcoming abuse offers peace. No longer will you be disquieted. You can be free. Accept His peace today.

> **"For you shall go out with joy, And be led out with peace."**
> **Isaiah 55:12**

BASILIA'S STORY

RICK AND I MET while we were both serving in the military overseas. We were both fresh out of college. I was deployed and assigned to the same mission he was. Rick initiated conversation with me whenever our paths crossed, although he appeared to blush and gave me shy smiles. As he increasingly got my attention, he would make flirtatious compliments about my appearance. Rick said he was mesmerized by my beauty and asked me out on a date. I had just broken up with a fella (a pharmacist) that had come on too strong and was proposing before I could even develop some feelings or chemistry for him! Worst of all, he said that I didn't even have to work if I didn't want to; I could be a homemaker. Rick and I fell in love within the first three months of dating and announced our engagement to our parents long-distance over the phone. Rick didn't want to wait to return to the U.S. to get married—he thought it would be exciting to marry overseas, and I agreed with him.

We put on our Sunday best and got married through the Justice of the Peace. It wasn't until after that (while we were making arrangements for our church wedding) that I found out that Rick had been married before. I grew up in the Greek Orthodox Church, and when we went to see a priest to marry us, he wouldn't marry us because Rick had been divorced and he wasn't Greek Orthodox; he said the Holy Synod (committee of Bishops) would not approve of our marriage. Rick was basically unchurched and claimed no particular religion; he said his parents had visited so many different types of churches when he was a child, he didn't know *what* religion to claim!

We proceeded to make arrangements with a military Protestant chaplain who agreed to marry us. I also found out from Rick during our church wedding planning that he did not want me to invite his parents because they were in the process of getting a divorce after thirty years of marriage. I had already told Rick that if we married overseas, my parents and family wouldn't be able to attend because they could not afford the trip while they were still raising my nine siblings back home. Within the first six months of meeting, we had a small military church wedding with just our friends as guests. It was a military wedding but quite untraditional as I was not given away; I walked down the aisle alone wearing a pink wedding dress. I had elected to wear pink, even though it was my first time getting married, because it was Rick's second marriage. Go figure, what was I thinking? I was *already hooked* into always adapting to his comfort zone, ignoring and compromising my own identity and needs.

Everything went well, and we had some romantic dating adventures before the wedding. It was on our honeymoon night that Rick and I had our first quarrel. We were on a cruise ship. Rick had gotten in a lousy mood during dinner and steadily declined into a nit-picky disposition. Everything I said was somehow misunderstood. Prior to this, I was able to talk freely about my dreams and aspirations regarding school and children in the future, but suddenly there was a dark, negative, disapproving remark interjected into every part of my conversation with him. I lost my appetite, and he demanded that I finish my meal. Rick said we weren't leaving the table until I finished. Here I was all dressed up during a romantic evening that I had so looked forward to, and my eyes were welled-up with tears. I couldn't even see my food, let alone swallow it! I had a huge lump in my throat. My feelings were shattered. It felt like my heart had been cut into; I ached so badly. How could he love me and act this way on our honeymoon?

I wondered if he had drunk too much. But he had drunk wine, beer, or champagne when we were dating, and he had not become argumentative like now. Usually when he drank alcohol, he would just be relaxed and mellow (or become obnoxiously silly or jolly). That night when we went back to our honeymoon suite and I asked Rick why he was being moody and so hateful toward me, he became *livid*! Rick slapped me across the face, yelling, "I am not being hateful!" I began to cry as he had slapped me hard enough that I had lost my balance and landed by our suitcase. My eye had hit the corner of the luggage stand, and he quickly came over, kissed my face, and started crying, begging me to forgive him. I was so very much in love with him, I was quick to forgive. We made up.

This was not the end of Rick's erratic mood changes. Rick would go for periods of time and be the greatest guy to hang out with as a husband and friend, but then he would get upset about the smallest things, like when the kitchen cupboards weren't the way that he had organized them. If I moved the canned goods unknowingly while I cooked meals, he would be irate to find that the cans weren't in the order that he had set them! After a while, it seemed like Rick was unhappy about *anything* I said or did; the food, laundry, or cleaning wasn't being done correctly. Rick would complain, and his gnawing complaining usually led to a huge argument. It never failed that on the most special events or holidays, he would start up with his fussing and grumbling. It was like he couldn't allow us to be happy during special times—instead, he would be extremely dissatisfied with something.

One Christmas, while we were still serving overseas, he got into a melancholy mood after hanging up the phone with his mother. I had overheard him arguing with her. So I gently asked him, "Is everything okay back home?" Rick *snapped* and pushed me against the wall (knocking over our living room lamp and breaking it) while yelling at my face, "That is none of your business!" Rick had what I thought to be an unusual relationship with his mother. They argued over the phone constantly. Yet, whenever he pulled night guard duty, she would call him in the morning to give him a wakeup call to check that he had heard his alarm! She never called him "Rick." Up until this day, she still calls him by his name as a boy: "Ricky." I told him that night that I couldn't take his temper and his hurting me anymore. I told him I was leaving him; he told me that he was very sorry and that he would never hurt me that way again. I told him that I needed some time to think about it, and he got mad again and shouted, "If you leave, I want all of the Christmas gifts I gave you back!" I left Rick for a week and stayed with some military friends. During that time, I talked to the chaplain that married us. I told him how depressed I was with Rick, that we argued all the time, and about his constant belittling of me and even *hitting* me. The chaplain said that I needed to forgive him and start over. So, I went back to him when he called me at my friends', pleading for me to forgive him.

Before we completed our overseas assignment, I found out that I was pregnant. The medical personnel were so excited for me! But when I came home to tell Rick the news, he said he wasn't ready to have children. Rick convinced me that we were both too young to start a family and that we should spend some time as a couple first before becoming parents. After all, he said, we had only been married a year! I was very disappointed and

BASILIA'S STORY

lost my excitement about the baby when Rick suggested that I have an abortion (because we could always have children later in our marriage). I knew *nothing* at that time about pregnancy or that there was an actual baby in my womb. I was told by Rick and the medical staff at the clinic that it was just tissue that would be scraped from my uterus and not an actual baby. I couldn't call my parents to discuss my situation because they hadn't even discussed the facts of life with me as a teenager!

Sex was never talked about in my family. I received all of my sex education from peers along the way. My parents had a loving relationship. Although they were good parents, they were both overly protective and strict with my siblings and me. For example, we were allowed friends to visit us, but we couldn't visit their homes. Perhaps they were so overprotective because we lived in such a large city—full of what most cities are like. Maybe it was their culture, the way they were raised in their Greek ancestry. Whenever we siblings were faced with challenges, our parents' smothering separated us from reaching out to them. Rick became very supportive of me when I complied with his request to wait to have a baby. All I wanted at this point was not to argue with him so that he wouldn't keep losing his temper. I wanted us to go back to the loving, romantic relationship that we shared while we were dating. My heart was empty and full of grief. On one of those sad, heartbreaking days while I was on my lunch break, I stopped at a bookstore to distract myself. While browsing, I thought about the fact that I had begun to struggle with my weight. I realize now that it was just my body changing into a young woman and that I had to learn that I could no longer eat the same empty calorie foods that I used to eat. Nevertheless, I had gained fifteen pounds, and though I carried it well because I am tall, I was miserable! Rick never even noticed as I didn't look overweight. I had started to do some binging and purging (I felt guilty for being overweight), so I used laxatives to get rid of my meals whenever I overate. I was dealing with bulimia. I was so depressed over Rick and *now* this ordeal with myself!

While at this bookstore, I picked up a book that I now know was a devotional, but I bought it thinking it was an inspirational poetry book. Within that book, I found the plan of salvation—the invitation! Later, while all alone, I asked for God's forgiveness of my sins and for Him to come into my heart. I no longer felt a desire to return to the Greek Orthodox Church. I had always had a discomfort as a child with the rituals that I was taught and expected to abide by. I now had this *personal relationship* with *God*. All I wanted to do now was what this devotional book said I could do, and that was to worship Him, not priests, bishop committees, or saints. It said, just like in the Bible, that I could go *directly* to Christ in prayer with all of my praises, hurts, questions, and needs for comfort and guidance. I didn't tell Rick about my newfound relationship with God as I knew now that sharing my thoughts and feelings only brought about a brawl.

Our enlistment terms of service in the military ended about the same time and because we both wanted to enroll in medical school, I decided not to re-enlist. Rick wanted to re-enlist and said he would register to take night classes while waiting to be accepted into medical school. I had already applied and had gotten accepted. This was a rosy period for me. I had prayed for God's deliverance from my bulimia and had received the strength to manage my eating habits into eating nutritiously. This ultimately led to my returning to my normal weight. God was faithful in drawing me out of that vicious bulimic cycle—I was healed by His mercy. Rick was in what appeared to be remission from his bouts of fits. Perhaps he was just happy about the idea of soon being able to return to the States.

After our discharge from the military we decided to move to Rick's hometown of Belmont, California. I was raised in Los Angeles, California, so I was not used to living in a suburban

BASILIA'S STORY

area at all. I found a job quickly as a physician's assistant (due to my experience in the military). I was very excited about being back in school, but it soon became a nightmare! Rick didn't want me driving to school alone, so he demanded that I schedule my classes around his schedule so we could ride together. This was difficult because some of my classes were not being taught on the days that he had his classes. It became even more difficult—extremely difficult—when he began a pattern of picking a fight on the drive to school! I was so stressed out and crying most of the time on our drives. I was also struggling with my concentration in classes.

Rick would occasionally ask me to write his class papers for him since I had already taken some of the classes he was taking. This was very annoying because he got "A" grades for my work, and I had to take time away from my studies to do his. But I did it to keep the peace; he would become very volatile if I declined to help him with his class papers. Just as I was getting very close to completing all of my core classes, Rick said that he didn't want me to go to school anymore and that he forbade me to continue. I was devastated and got into a heated argument with him, which ended with him driving home recklessly and throwing things around *and* at me when we got home. I was so frightened, I felt my knees knocking while my body felt frozen, not knowing how I was going to get away from his attack on me. I reached out for the landline phone, and he said, "Get away from that phone; you're not calling anyone orgoing *anywhere!*" Rick unplugged the phone from the wall.

I kept asking Rick why he was so upset and what I had possibly done to make him so furious; he eventually yelled out that on that day, he had been thinking about his ex-wife and how he had hurt her and that this had upset him. Rick shared that the reason for his divorce was not what he had told me. Rick had told me that they just couldn't get along and that she divorced him because she didn't love him anymore. Rick then said, "I cheated on her and hit her just like I've hit you." Rick cried like a baby and said he was so sorry about her and that she had re-married and had gotten killed (shot in the head) by the man she married. Rick then told me that he grew up around arguing; he said that his father used to hit his mother and his siblings. Rick added that he hadn't told me this while dating because he was afraid I wouldn't marry him. Rick asked if I could forgive him for losing his temper that day; he then wanted to hug, snuggle, and go to bed. My heart was so heavy. I hurt so badly the next morning as I drove my *exhausted self* back to work. I dreaded the thought of going back to school that night and what Rick would be like.

Rick didn't stop me from going to school that night; instead, he announced that he was dropping out of med school and that he planned on finishing but that right now he just wanted to do his military Reserves duty so he could draw a good retirement pension someday. By this time, Rick's parents had divorced and both had re-married. Things were going well again, and his birthday was coming up. I wanted to surprise him with a gift. I called my mother-in-law on a Saturday while Rick was at work and asked her if she would like to join me for lunch and accompany me to get Rick's birthday present. We had such a good girl time! I was so excited to get Rick a shirt, which he had looked at recently and had said he liked the pattern and would love to have it.

That birthday evening, I had prepared a candlelight dinner and had romantic music playing when he arrived. Everything was good until I handed him his birthday gift. Rick opened it and looked up at me in a rage; he said it had to go back to the store and that he didn't want it! Rick was yelling at the top of his lungs; he kept repeating that how dare I go to town behind his back! I reassured him that I had purchased the shirt with my own birthday money that my family had sent me. Rick said, "It doesn't

BASILIA'S STORY

matter; it's still going back!" Rick was squeezing my arms and talking into my face when he said that. I told him he was hurting me, and he said, "Too bad, you're the one that messed up!" and he squeezed me even harder. I had bruised arms and wore long sleeves to cover them up the next few days.

It was at this point that I began to realize that *no matter what I did* to make things better in our home life, nothing was changing. Doing all the cooking, laundry, and cleaning *just right* on top of working at the clinic and going to school wasn't improving Rick's mood or our marriage. Worst of all, I began to notice that my car tires were frequently marked with white chalk. At first, I thought it was the meter police from school, but then while I was looking for a pen in a drawer, I found some chalk that I had not purchased. I also found some sticky notes hidden under some papers with what looked like speedometer readings from my car. I only knew this because Rick's car was new; he would trade his cars in every year (he always had low mileage). The mileage on his sticky notes matched closer to my speedometer. It was then that I realized that he was keeping track of my coming and going from school and errands.

There was a co-worker that approached me with a concerned look and asked me how things were going at home. For the first time, I confided in someone outside of my family. She asked me if Rick was being abusive toward me. When I said, "yes," she invited me to stay in her guest room at her home for as long as I needed to. Her husband was in the military, and she worked part-time at the clinic with me. I took her up on her offer. I talked to Rick the next day after another one of his explosive episodes where he had attempted to lock me in the house (because I had inquired as to why he didn't call to say he wouldn't be home for dinner, and I asked about the chalk and speedometer readings).

I had fixed dinner as usual the previous night, but Rick had been a no-show for dinner; it was two in the morning when he got home. Rick had responded with, "Shut up, I don't have to answer to you!" Apparently, he had been drinking and smelled of booze and perfume. I had called the police after he grabbed me by the arm (as I headed for the door). I used my other hand to grab the phone and dialed 911, yelling, "Police, please!" The police were able to track our phone number to our residence, but what followed was unbelievable (and something I have never forgotten)! Rick managed to appear coherent in the presence of the police officers who arrived five minutes after my call. Rick smiled and said, "I'm sorry, officers, I guess we got carried away with our arguing. We really do love each other. We're sorry we disturbed the peace. We do like our neighbors." One officer looked over at me as I was sobbing and in obvious distress and said, "You two need to work things out and get some counseling. We're cops; we don't get involved in domestic arguments. That's *not* our job." I said, "But officer, he was being rough with me, and I'm afraid if I stay here, he's going to hurt me." The officer said, "Then get a restraining order. Without *that*, I can't restrict him from you; he's your husband!"

So, my friend's offer for a place *to think things through* came at a time where I was at a loss for what to do! Women had been calling our home, asking for Rick. When I had asked him who they were, he said it was none of my business but that if I had to know, he had met them while on military assignments, and they were the ones calling *him* and *he* wasn't calling *them*. As if that made it right—how did they get our home number? Rick had to have given it to them! Our episode with the police, and the women's phone calls were the reasons I used to tell Rick that I was going to take some "time out" from the relationship. I was shocked that he agreed to the temporary separation, and he said that he really wanted for us not to break up, that maybe it would be good for us to be apart to work out our relationship. I asked if he would go to counseling with me during the separation, and he agreed to.

I stayed at my friend's home, worked, and went to counseling with Rick two times per week. By then, I had put school temporarily on hold because I was so confused; I was experiencing so much lack of sleep, worrying about our relationship and not being able to get my class readings done. We were separated for six months, and things got better in our counseling sessions. Rick made a commitment to talk to me in a normal tone and not to physically hurt me. I moved back in, but not even an entire day had passed when he was back to reversing whatever I said to him. It was as if he had to have something to be picky about, something to argue about and to blame me for. Rick couldn't allow himself or me to have a good day. I felt so discouraged. I didn't have an ounce of energy left within me.

I resigned and proceeded to give my four-week notice at work. I couldn't continue to help people at the clinic when I desperately needed help myself. I decided to apply for every academic scholarship available to go back to school full-time. I felt that I could do well in school if I could make it my full-time job but that I couldn't deal with work, school, and Rick's mistreatment all at once. In the meantime, something unexpected happened. My birth control pills failed me *again*. I got pregnant. Perhaps I had failed to maintain regular, healthy patterns of rest in the midst of the overwhelming stress that I was carrying, and the pills couldn't work their course. I don't know. Although I was surprised and weary, I experienced the joy that only a first-time mother can ever experience.

I told Rick, and he was angrier than I had *ever* seen him! Rick said, "I told you I'm not ready to be a parent! Get rid of it; it's probably not even mine!" Rick brushed harshly past me, threw a laundry basket at me, which knocked me over when I attempted to duck. If ever I had hurt, this was the day that he killed my love for him. Rick had managed to kill my soul! How could he allege that I had been with another man? I had *never* been unfaithful to him. Rick's the one that had even slept with my best friend in med school!

I asked if we could go back to counseling, and he agreed. In counseling, I let him know that I was going to have our baby, and he said he wanted a paternity test. I agreed to his request even though it was humiliating, and I was deeply offended. I felt totally oppressed by his pressure for the test. Rick said he wanted a divorce and that he didn't want to be married anymore. Rick said that it was either the baby or him. I said that I would be moving out and told him that I chose our baby; he went ballistic in the counseling session. Rick said, "Just so you know, I'm not going to pay you child support!" The therapist—to my shock—did not confront him on his lack of anger control or inappropriateness toward me. Instead, he said that in view of Rick's decision to end the marriage that we would not be meeting for counseling as a couple anymore. I asked the counselor if he would be willing to testify in court during the divorce proceedings. The counselor said, "No—that would be a conflict of interest." Rick had been the one to hire our marriage counselor. Rick wanted the divorce, but he refused to pay for it, so I had to file and pay for it. I couldn't believe it. We had been married for eight years and I was pregnant, and Rick wanted a divorce! I was distraught and in such despair. I began to notice that I would have an unexpected vision of taking a knife to my wrist; my own thoughts scared me, and I pushed the vision away.

At the court hearing, Rick negotiated with his attorney and mine that if I were to drop the reason for the divorce from "domestic violence" to "incompatibility," he would pay a small amount of child support. My attorney met with his attorney and the judge in private quarters to request that in return, I would be given full custody of our unborn child in view of the fact that

BASILIA'S STORY

Rick had already assaulted me while pregnant and had raped me during our marriage. The reason for the divorce was changed to "incompatibility" so it wouldn't hurt Rick's employment record. I got full custody of our baby, but Rick was not ordered any child support because he pleaded on the stand that he was planning to go back to medical school and that he needed his income to pay for that; whereas, I had a full academic scholarship for med school and a grant to work part-time. Therefore, supposedly I was gainfully employed. Rick was allowed to manipulate his way out of child support. I thanked my attorney after the court hearing, and he said, "What for? I didn't do anything for you." One thing that was helpful to me and meant a lot was that my pastor offered to be at the court house and to wait for me until the hearing was over. My pastor did not make it, but he sent his sweet young-adult daughter, who prayed with me and was there with me in his place.

I believe that my source of strength kicked in when that one co-worker offered supportive guidance (and her home as temporary shelter). It seemed like right after that, I began to meet other friends that encouraged me through church, Bible study, and Christian women's club. I had my baby—a baby boy. I rededicated my life to Christ, and my close relationship to Him transformed every decision I have made ever since. Rick knew by now that God had become my source of strength and direction; he mocked me and said angrily that we didn't have anything in common anymore because I no longer drank, smoked, or cussed like him (or all he had imposed upon me to say or do). Going through med school, being an intern, and raising an infant into a healthy child *all at the same time* was only made possible because of *His power* within me.

Rick never went back to med school; he retired from the Reserves. Five years after I graduated from med school, I met my current husband, Seth, at the hospital that I was working at. Seth was single and different than any other man that I had dated. It was apparent that he was a godly man. Seth expressed an unconditional love for me, which I had never experienced before. Plus, my son became very fond of him. When Seth proposed, he offered to adopt my son. We got engaged the first year that we dated and married nine months later. It was a very special wedding because we were united in Christ, and I truly felt like I was getting married for the very first time in my life. We had an elegant, traditional wedding (yes, I wore a beautiful ivory bridal gown), and all of our family members and close friends attended.

I am blessed that I had already raised my son in the Lord as a single parent and that in spite of his broken family from infancy through childhood, he is a healthy, successful Christian man today. Seth and I have been married for twenty-five years now. We are supportive of one another's medical careers and have raised a family centered on God's love. Seth and I have two daughters of our own. They are both on their way to becoming Proverbs 31 women. Rick never allowed Seth to adopt my son, but my son considers Seth as his father and has always called him "Dad," just like our daughters. We have four grandchildren from my son, and every now and then, Rick will still bad mouth me to our son or grandchildren. Rick has attempted to do the same with Seth. However, Rick has learned that Seth does not give merit to his negative talk about me, so his derogatory remarks to Seth have gradually faded away.

My first marriage was like being constantly tortured and not knowing why. I was always confused about Rick's lip talk that he loved me, and yet his actions showed otherwise. Life with Rick was packed with unpredictable turmoil and feeling low about myself. I reached a state of depression where I was so lethargic that I had trouble getting up in the mornings. I had no energy, not even to make my own cup of coffee (I skipped the coffee, got it at the office, or drove through to get it). It's a pleasantry to make my coffee in the morning nowadays! I regret that I didn't end my relationship with Rick early on—I lost some of the best years of my life. Instead of tolerating the abuse, breaking up, and making up so many times, I should have ended the relationship because this only hindered my spirit and increased the years that I was trapped in the relationship!

My life since I ended my relationship with Rick is focused on being right with God and not being right with Rick or any other humankind. I no longer have an empty place in my heart with desperation as to what terrible things are going to happen to me next in my marriage. My life is full of ease and faith in the present and future. There is no fear that I will *ever* return to an abusive relationship. I am so done with that! I live a life of gratitude now; I am fulfilled. My heart has healed. I have His peace.

PART IV

ENCOURAGEMENT FOR THE VICTIM & *OVERCOMER*

You Shall Overcome and be Led Out with Peace
I WANT TO ENCOURAGE you to *never* give up your freedom for abuse. Suffice it to say that it has been my privilege and experience to work with so many victims that began their journey from the dark pit of their abuse and now live an illuminated *Overcomer* life worth living. There is no honor in staying imprisoned as a victim. A victim may have said "I do" to her abuser, but there comes a time when she reaches a perspective that she *knows* she's being abused, and she now has to say, "I don't" to the abuser and the abuse. That's when she enters the path of an *Overcomer*.

These books have covered the subject of abuse and family violence extensively, and much has been shared on exposing the abuser. This emphasis is my gift to *you* who are being abused because my desire is for you to know how very special you are before the Lord. My last word of encouragement is for you to be encouraged and to be an encourager. To encourage is an act of love. Being an encourager means having a generosity of spirit. The only way a victim can begin to give away the love she has been given by God is if she has fully accepted her *Overcomer* role and the potency of His Love which she has received. God's love, and everything we receive, is by grace alone. God's love can never be paid back, but it can be paid onward by choosing to pattern after Him and by encouraging others in His love. He has summoned you through His Holy Spirit to become a willing instrument of His love, reflecting His peace unto the discouraged. Philippians 2:4 instructs us, "Let each of you look out not only for his own interests, but also for the interests of others." Following the instructions in this verse can lead to the healing of the traumatic wounds of a victim.

If you come alongside a victim and encourage her, it gives her courage to become an *Overcomer*. In order to enter the lifestyle of an *Overcomer*, a victim must rise to the *Overcomer* challenge: To hide God's Word in her heart, live in peace, live the victorious life, and allow the *Overcomer* principles to become her arsenal. The challenge to be encouraged and become an encourager not only readies you for your own mission as an *Overcomer*, but it also prepares you to witness to victims of abuse by using the *Overcomer* offensive and defensive weapons with which you have been equipped. Through the empowerment of the Holy Spirit, *Overcomers* receive the strength and authority to serve victims and to re-build them for His Kingdom. Encourage a victim; He will use your renewed strength mightily! An *Overcomer* has learned the meaning of the verses in Matthew 25:35-40 when Christ speaks to His apostles about having compassion for others in their time of need; He said that when we help those that are hurting, it is the same as doing it to Him.

ENCOURAGEMENT FOR THE VICTIM & OVERCOMER

An *Overcomer*'s compassion serves victims through His love. An *Overcomer* naturally becomes an agent of change for victims and future generations.

The introduction of this book made reference to Jesus as your good Shepherd. That makes you one of His lambs. The Scriptures call Jesus Himself the Lamb of God. A lamb in biblical days was a highly valued possession. The Bible tells us that before God sent Jesus to Earth, it was a religious tradition to offer a lamb as a sacrifice for the forgiveness of sin. You don't need to offer yourself as a sacrificial lamb by tolerating abuse as this does not provide peace—nor does it fulfill the common good. Jesus has *already* been the sacrificial lamb for the entire human race. He is indeed your good Shepherd, but He does not intend for you to become a sacrificial lamb. He is your protector—your Father-Shepherd!

My hope is that you were able to identify in some way with the longsuffering experienced by the former victims who shared their stories and that although overcoming their abuse was not easily and magically accomplished, you may have gained insight as to what it's going to take for *you* to overcome your abuse. In addition, I hope this book has prompted you to seek wisdom and counsel from those that are trained and experienced in the treatment of abuse. C.S. Lewis said, "The next best thing to being wise oneself is to live in a circle of those who are." Proverbs 1:5-6a states "A wise man will hear and increase learning, and a man of understanding will attain wise counsel, to understand a proverb and an enigma."

An abuser may pride himself on being an enigma, but a victim can learn to peel off his camouflage. The *Overcomers* that were presented in this book are *courageous* women who were all involved in the downward spiral of abusive relationships. At some point in their life, they each decided that they could no longer tolerate and accept their unhealthy relationship. Today, they are triumphant *Overcomers*. They were as devastated as you are today, but now they are destined to live joyous, *peaceful* lives! He, alone, has the power to vanquish your ugly past abuse and to turn it into something beautiful. Christ sees and views all of us as divinely lovely in His sight, however underdeveloped we are; He takes each of us and molds us into a beautifully refined, purposeful being. Your Heavenly Father goes beyond the pattern you've followed in your life; He sees His entire objective as He molds you into who He created you to be. The Lord receives a victim into His Hands and molds her into a unique *Overcomer*.

The Bible has over thirty verses with figurative examples of how God is our Maker—the Potter—and we are the clay. In a nutshell, the message in these verses is this: We have the choice to become who He molds us to be and to take the road He has carved out and ordained for us—or not. What is fundamental in a relationship with God is not what you do for Him, but rather what you consent for Him to do with you (transform you and your life). Are you willing to allow Him to mold you, and will you choose to walk on the path He has designed for you to take? When you live in communion with your Lord and Savior and follow the precepts and wisdom He provides, nothing can stop your journey of joy, your development, nor dispel your peace of mind.

Right now, you may feel discouraged and tempted to give up trying to fight away the abuse in your life. Discouragement is one of satan's most fun weapons to throw at you; he is your adversary. When you reject your abuse, he will attempt to use others to thwart your efforts. satan's only plan is to devalue you and God and to minimize your relationship with Him. Do not get discouraged. Fight discouragement by praying and asking that God's will be revealed to you. Move forward confidently, knowing that God will be with you and will lead you into whatever His will is for your life. If you're still feeling a wee bit discouraged and lacking in hope—even after reading the women's testimo-

ENCOURAGEMENT FOR THE VICTIM & OVERCOMER

nies in this book—turn to the books of the Bible, especially Philippians and Colossians. Those books were written while Paul was on house arrest.

If your mind keeps wondering if the *Overcomer* journey is worth the trip, know emphatically that your *Overcomer* destination is worth the entire trip! God's all-embracing love and peace is able to encircle and touch every facet of your journey from being victimized to overcoming your abuse. Read Paul's book of Ephesians; it's one of the greatest tonics for anyone who's discouraged and ailing in hope. Becoming an *Overcomer* is going to require you to become more introspective and honest about yourself and your abusive relationship; it will take time to educate yourself on abuse both academically and spiritually. It will entail being willing to do *whatever* is healthy and *everything* that is necessary to end the abuse. A victim is simply idling—be productive and draw up an *Overcomer* to-do list. Ask yourself, "What about *me*? Am *I* willing to surrender *my* abuse? Or, would I rather remain oppressed? Do I want me and my future generations to remain captive for the rest of our lives?"

My questions may sound rather callous or harsh, but I want to love you enough to point out the risks of avoiding the needed changes in your life. A family system is the essence of a society and a nation as a whole. Families impact *everyone* in positive and negative ways. Families can introduce healthy bonding, love, nurturance, and personal growth; or, they can influence the learning of destructive patterns of behavior. Truth be known, a marital or family argument does not have to turn into a fatality. Please don't misunderstand me to be saying that marriages and families shouldn't ever have intense arguments. I'm saying that learning to work together to communicate and interact appropriately and productively is critical in the process of acquiring healthy relationships.

Marriages and families do not have to agree on every issue; we can still accept and love the other even if their personality or way of thinking seems odd. We have discussed in earlier pages that there are no perfect parents and no perfect children. Based on that telling observation, we can deduce that there are no perfect families. All families have descended from our disobedient first parents and their family written about in Genesis 3 and 4. Adam and Eve are our spiritual ancestors; they bore the first family. The most respected families in our communities have experienced what happened in the Garden of Eden: manipulation, lying, rebellion, disloyalty, betrayal, relationship breakdowns, murder, death, deceit, hurt, disappointment, broken rules, consequences, and a longing for unconditional love and peace.

On moral issues, if there are established boundaries, there is *no reason* for constant disagreements on limits that have already been set. If there's doubt and differences on moral issues, search the Bible together for answers. There are no problem-solving resolutions to be had with married couples or families shouting at the top of their lungs about how bad or wrong someone has been. There is *no peace* in chaotic marital and destructive family relationships. Isaiah 51:11b-12a reassures you that, "They shall obtain joy and gladness; Sorrow and sighing shall flee away. 'I, *even* I, *am* He who comforts you.'" Take a moment to pause *right now* and say out loud, "*You* are an anointed daughter of the King of the Universe—He has called *you* to *joy* and to *peace* to be more than a conqueror—an *Overcomer!*" Try Him out, and you shall have not only His comfort but also His joy and His *peace!*

If at the moment you're feeling sorrow over your abusive relationship and your family. Ask yourself, "Am I able to establish and acquire healthy family relationships while living in an abusive relationship?"

Let it be known to you *without a shadow of a doubt* that if God has placed in your heart the desire to live an abuse-free life, then

ENCOURAGEMENT FOR THE VICTIM & OVERCOMER

it is sealed with His Will and approval and desire for your life! Some misunderstand the Scripture in Psalm 37:4, "Delight yourself also in the LORD, And He shall give you the desires of your heart," to mean that God will give you *whatever your heart desires*. This completely skips the part that it is God *Himself* through the power of the Holy Spirit who places within our heart any good desires with His purpose for our life. *He* is the One that gives you the desires of your heart! And, He is the only One Who through the power of the Holy Spirit can let you know His Will for your life. "For it is God who works in you both to will and to do for *His* good pleasure" (Philippians 2:13).

We have discussed how God is an unfailing God; He has never failed, so by becoming an *Overcomer*, you will not fail. Being made in His Image means that just like He is One with Christ and Spirit, you are also one with God. His Spirit lives within you. Each time God lovingly gazes at you, He sees His Son within you. There can be no peace or joyous harmony while living in dread and fear. Faith births God within, which then breeds security and joy—producing peace within. The God within you has *already* overcome. His Spirit and desire to overcome has already been placed in your heart. It is a *green light*. GO!

This book extols the virtues of establishing a functional, loving relationship; it promotes healthy, functional family living. Not because it's acquired easily—but because when you decide to work on a functional family system, it *does* bring peace. Notice I said *work* on a healthy family system; that's because all relationships take work. But fear not, you don't have to go at it alone. You have an *awesome* God to help you accomplish that! In the New King James Version of the Bible, the word *awesome* is used twenty-three times to describe God—and that's because He is *all that* and then some! *Awesome* is meant to convey "inspiring awe." The word *awesome* was originally used exclusively to describe God and His works of awe. His Works in your life as an

Overcomer are indeed awesome! Here are a few of those Scriptures to encourage you:

> "Come and see the works of God; *He is* awesome *in His* doing toward the sons of men" (Psalm 66:5).

> "O God, *You* are more awesome than Your holy places. The God of Israel *is* He who gives strength and power to *His* people" (Psalm 68:35).

> "You shall not be terrified of them; for the LORD your God, the great and awesome God, *is* among you" (Deuteronomy 7:21).

> "And He said: "Behold, I make a covenant. Before all your people I will do marvels such as have not been done in all the earth, nor in any nation; and all the people among whom you *are* shall see the work of the LORD. For it *is* an awesome thing that I will do with you" (Exodus 34:10).

> "And I looked, and arose and said to the nobles, to the leaders, and to the rest of the people, 'Do not be afraid of them. Remember the Lord, great and awesome, and fight for your brethren, your sons, your daughters, your wives, and your houses'" (Nehemiah 4:14).

In Luke 4:18, Jesus said: "The Spirit of the LORD *is* upon Me, because He has anointed Me to preach the gospel to the poor. He has sent Me to heal *the* brokenhearted, to proclaim liberty to *the* captives And recovery of sight to *the* blind, *To* set at liberty those who are oppressed." Do you want to be free in your

ENCOURAGEMENT FOR THE VICTIM & OVERCOMER

spirit? Do you truly want to experience His peace? Jesus often helped and healed those with physical illnesses, but when He ministered deliverance to the captives and recovered sight for the blind, His ministry included spiritual application in these areas. Sin, as foremost, is the oppressive foundation that blinds us and condemns us to be bound into the blind bondage of sin against ourselves and God. When Jesus saw the woman at the well (John 4), He saw a woman who was thirsty and yearning for genuine love and acceptance. Mostly, He saw a human being who was void of what only He could give—peace in her heart. Becoming an *Overcomer is* a total worthwhile makeover and faith lift. Like with the woman at the well, becoming an *Overcomer* is a spiritual makeover. It is a transfiguration!

You, too, can have that kind of peace in your heart because, like with the woman at the well, Christ does not have second-class standards for a victim of abuse—only first-class *Overcomer* standards! Your Creator God, the One that has the power that no one on Earth has the equivalent to give you (that *peace* in your heart), loves you mightily! He's gazing at you right now. Will you look at Him? It's comforting to know that He's watching over you lovingly, but to directly look at Him—to look into Jesus' eyes—can be transfixing for your heart! Would you be willing to reciprocate His gaze and love today? Once you do it will transfigure you and your life.

Begin loving Him back by reading His Word. God's Word *is* God (John 1:1). When you open up the Bible, you are, in essence, turning to and listening to God. His Word is Truth: "The entirety of Your word *is* truth" (Psalm 119:160); "And you shall know the truth, and the truth shall make you free" (John 8:32). A victim plus God's Word is a potent combo—a powerful force! God and His Word-Power can solidify your peaceful walk with Him. Believe that He is the provider of *all* of your needs; after all, He *is* Jehovah-Jireh, Hebrew for: "The-Lord-Will-Provide"

(Genesis 22:14). He will provide you with courage and equip you with peace: "Peace I leave with you, My peace I give to you; not as the world gives do I give to you. Let not your heart be troubled, neither let it be afraid" (John 14:27).

He will even provide you with *Overcomer* scruples so you can move forward peacefully. Try as you may to justify your abuse, the only evaluation necessary as to whether you ought to allow abuse to have its way with you is to think about what the outcome of that abuse will be. Christ is the healer of all broken hearts; He is the supernatural glue Who sutures your brokenness. Are you willing to accept Jesus' mission to heal your broken heart and deliver you from captivity and oppression? In Luke 4, after Jesus concluded His message of deliverance from captivity, verse 21 reads, "And He began to say to them, *'Today this Scripture is fulfilled in your hearing.'*" How will *you* put into action everything that you have heard and learned from God's Word regarding Jesus's mission for your life? He has said in His Word that He came to deliver you from captivity; such a statement of grace and mercy with a promise of delivery from your oppression demands a response of faith from you as a victim and a response of faith from all of Jesus' hearers. Once you get a sip and a taste and experience Christ's Truth setting you free, the deliverance and peace you receive is too great to go back! Won't you RSVP to Christ's invitation to His Truth and His Peace with no regrets?

Within *Overcoming Abuse: Embracing Peace* Volume I and II, there are some aids for ending your victim role and claiming the life of an *Overcomer*, but they are certainly not an exhaustive set of failsafe encyclopedias. If *anything at all* was learned from these books, my hope is that you captured *Christ's message of His love that never fades away and that your identity and purpose for your life is in Him.* I pray that you've come to find out that He cares for you more than anything else in this world. His caring is

ENCOURAGEMENT FOR THE VICTIM & OVERCOMER

ineffable. He's your Friend and Companion. Shake His Hand and embrace the comfort of His consoling Arms from now on and for all of your days. His love for you is unmeasured and cannot be encompassed in the writings of these books; it goes above and beyond the scope of any book.

You, _____, were created to be an *Overcomer*. But please remember that the free will to be an *Overcomer* is nothing without the will to become one.

You have been offered a living hope that never expires and the gift of His merciful peace that is shielded by His power. If these books have instilled hope that you *can* overcome the abuse in your life and have cleared away the confusion that lives as a parasite in an abusive relationship, then they have *by grace* started your course to an abuse-free lifetime. If you've made a commitment to *overcome* your abuse and chosen *peace* in your life or have committed to help someone that's being abused, then these books have begun to fulfill their purpose. Thank you again for allowing me the time, for just a little while, to till the soil of your life and the privilege to plant a seed for the groundwork of an abused heart.

God bless you, *Overcomer*. God bless you, and your future generations, with freedom from abuse.

> **"The Lord bless you and keep you; The Lord make His face shine upon you, And be gracious to you; The Lord lift up His countenance upon you, And give you peace."**
> **Numbers 6:24-26**

CAROL'S STORY

I MET TOM IN Oklahoma City. Several couples had gotten together, and we went out on a date to a local nightclub to dance. Tom was with his date, and I was with mine, who happened to be Tom's friend. They knew each other through the military. Tom was an officer that had just returned from serving in Vietnam and was about to be discharged; whereas his friend was just being deployed to Vietnam. I was a senior in college. I visited with Tom that evening, but that was because we were sitting nearby. Tom called me several weeks later (he had gotten my phone number from his friend), and we went out to eat. I remember he treated me very nicely. I was especially interested in him because I was very much *of the world* and *materialistic* back then; he was apparently starting out real well, making good money with his work in sales!

I had not grown up *poor*-poor; I always had everything I needed. But I grew up in an area in Oklahoma where most of my friends had a lot more—and that's what I desired. Tom offered this, and that was kind of exciting to me. I know now that it's not right to have that much desire for the things of the world. I was flattered by him, and I was naïve; even though I had dated a lot, I was still naïve. After we dated for a couple of weeks, he told me that he was going to marry me! I responded with, "Oh yeah, right." Our relationship progressed, even while I was seeing a couple of other guys. One guy, I had dated for a year; he was pretty serious about me, maybe more than I was. As I look back, both of those guys that I had dated before Tom would have been better choices for me.

I had met Tom during the summer, and three weeks later, he talked about marriage. Tom never really did propose; we just went and looked at rings. Then, he gave me a ring that Christmas. Tom was Catholic but not a practicing Catholic; he didn't attend church. I had grown up in the Methodist church. Tom originally wanted to elope, which was okay with me, but my parents wanted us to have a church wedding. Tom had wanted to elope because he said people just have a big wedding to get gifts, and he could buy all of that! Tom did go ahead and talk to my dad. We married the next summer in the Methodist church.

All I knew about church was from the classes that I had attended. I just thought that if I died, I would automatically go to heaven because I was an okay person. I didn't know Jesus. My parents had five children, but they didn't raise us talking about the Bible or about our spiritual lives. My parents were in their forties before they really came to know Jesus; my brother got saved, and I believe he was the one to lead my parents to the Lord. My brother had been *into everything*; he had been the prodigal son. I was already married to Tom when I began to understand the gospel for the first time; it was actually about the same time that my parents understood it also.

Tom and I have two children—a daughter and son. We had been married three years when I got pregnant. I always wanted children, and he did not. But one day we were driving to Las Vegas and he said, "Throw your birth control pills out the window" *and I did*! I had been working as a teacher, but when I got pregnant, he wanted me to quit working—*so I did*. Right after that, he lost his job because he couldn't get along with the people in management. Here we were, both unemployed with no insurance and a new baby girl! When our daughter was nine months old, I learned that I was expecting again. Tom wasn't mad, but he was just okay with it. I thought that he would be thrilled when our son was born, because he would now have a son, but instead our son became his scapegoat. The way he treated him made me think that maybe our son *wasn't* welcome. It was obvious that our daughter was his favorite. Tom bonded with her early on; he was very punitive, ugly, and mean to our son.

People even noticed Tom's mistreatment of him. I can remember one of our neighbors commenting that she would hate to be Tom's son! Tom was *very* emotionally-abusive to our son and sometimes physically out of control. One time, I went over to Tom and told him to quit hurting him because he was going overboard. Tom could just lose it at any time, and you never knew when he was going to explode. Oftentimes I would think, "Why?" Tom came from a very dysfunctional family; both his parents were alcoholics and very manipulative. Tom's grandmother told me about the times that Tom's father would pull his sister's hair. I knew some of this before I married him, but these warning signs didn't affect me. Like I said, I was naïve. My thinking was that those were *his parents*. We've got our life over here, and we're going to be okay.

I actually should have known that *I* was being abused as early as our honeymoon. We were in the Caribbean, and there were a couple of single women traveling together which he invited to have dinner with us. I didn't say anything to him; I just allowed it to occur. The whole time during our honeymoon, he wouldn't spend any time with me. I would ask him to come to the pool with me, but he would rather be out on the putting green. I would go out there with him some of the time, but I just didn't get it; why would he rather spend time on his own? I felt hurt and rejected, but I didn't share my feelings because there was always this rage that erupted if I said anything. If I shared my feelings or had an opinion about something, he thought I was being critical of him. It was always an attitude of "that's *not* the way it's going to be—it's got to be my way." I knew that if there weren't other people around, he would lose his temper, that's for sure!

It was so gradual for me to determine that I was being abused by my husband. I knew that it wasn't right (and I also knew it wasn't something that had gone on in my home that I grew up in). Growing up in my family wasn't perfect by any means. We did have one problem—we didn't talk. So I didn't have much practice in expressing myself appropriately. My parents, siblings, and I did have meals together, but we never really had any meaningful conversations at the table. It's like we lived out our separate lives. We met for meals and didn't *really connect emotionally;* we just went our different ways after each meal. However, I did feel cared for and loved. I had a close relationship with my parents, especially with my dad. I felt very special, and I could visit with him. They had high aspirations for me; they were good parents.

Perhaps with Mom there could have been some mother-daughter rivalry, possibly; we got closer as I became an adult. My mom passed away, and my dad remarried. It was Dad that I went to when I figured out that I was in an abusive relationship. I would explain a little bit to him, but not totally. I told him that there was trouble, but I was really vague, and he would ask what I wanted to do. I would say, "I don't know." Dad told me that divorce brings on a lot more problems, and that I should think about that because he knew that Tom had an explosive temper. One thing that stood out in my mind that Dad said was, "Well, I don't know if you'll ever be able to stand up to Tom." When I thought about what he said to me, I said to myself, "Stand up to my husband. I never thought you had to stand up to your husband?!" I then thought, "Well, maybe you are supposed to." But, I wasn't mature enough or able to do it for the longest time, and then when I did, I did it wrong—I did it in anger.

My methods for dealing with conflict up until then were more or less to back off or to cry. That's what I had chosen to do with Tom. I had a problem-solving strategy of "What can *I do* to make it better?" I thought this way for a long, long time. Whenever we got into an argument, Tom would threaten me with a divorce; he knew I didn't want a divorce. For years, he constantly threatened so I would back off. Tom had convinced me that I couldn't make it on my own on a teacher's salary, which I believed back then because of the lifestyle that I had gotten used to—I know different and better now.

It wasn't until the kids were in elementary school that I realized that I shouldn't be in that abusive marriage! I was noticing the kids being hurt and not being treated properly. It was at this point that Tom threatened me again with a divorce, and I responded with, "You go ahead and get an attorney; we will both get attorneys," and he backed off and never mentioned it again! I called his manipulative bluff to control me.

By this time, Tom was not able to keep down a job because he would lose his businesses due to his criminal activity in the sales. I had to be a part of that activity—it was *fraud*. I never saw any of Tom's paychecks the whole time I was married to him. Tom got all of the bank statements and paid all of the bills—if they got paid. For the most part, he did do financially well. A friend once asked me if Tom was involved in selling drugs because she had noticed that he made a lot of money. Everyone just saw how successful he was. In reality, toward the end of our marriage, he was being subpoenaed by the court for fraud, and he had become clinically depressed.

During the divorce process, Tom had suggested that we didn't need to physically move out, but that we could just live separately in our home. Tom said that he would not hurt me and that I would be upstairs, and he would be downstairs. We did that for a while. My dad and stepmom were scared for me because they knew what had recently transpired with Tom. Finally, it dawned on me that we couldn't live in the same household; some of the same stuff was happening again! I left and moved into another house that we owned.

This house was located in an area which was far away from county police protection. One night, Tom got enraged and called to tell me that he was coming after me and that he was going to kill me (I was out there with my daughter and son). That night I made a really bad decision—one that I will always regret. It was very dark. I left, and I left the kids at the house. I was going to have to drive country roads and interstate in the dark. I didn't know where Tom was coming from or how he was coming (he had already threatened my life just a few weeks before).

In my mind, I was thinking if he catches the kids and me out on the road and if we have an accident trying to get away from him, I wouldn't want *that* for them. I really didn't think he would hurt them in this way, but I didn't know for sure. I went to my parent's home. My stepmom was very supportive; she had been through a bad divorce process, so she understood me. I did get the kids back in a couple of days (some neighbors helped me to get them back to my parent's home). Apparently, Tom had gone into a spell of deep depression and couldn't care for them after all.

Another day, he came by the house, and he was acting crazy; he was threatening to kill himself! That is the day that I knew I definitely had no choice—I had to *completely* leave him. When I told him that I was not going to let him commit suicide, that I was going to stop him and that he was not going to do it, he said,

"Oh no, you're not because I'll tie you up!" I attempted to leave when he said that, and he chased me to the car and grabbed me by the throat. I thought I would literally die then, but I managed to frantically get loose, and I kicked the car door on him, knocking him down, and I ran to a neighbor's house. I called my dad, and we went to pick up the kids from school.

At last, I made a decision to end the abusive marriage. Daddy took me to a *rotten* Christian attorney—someone from his church. Although he was a kind, caring man, he wasn't man enough to deal with my ex-husband. When Tom and I met with my attorney, my attorney would try to counsel us against the divorce by kneeling next to Tom's chair and saying, "Well, I think we have a failure to communicate here—so what do you need to say to her?" I thought to myself, "Yeah, we have failed to communicate, but there is much more than that going on in this marriage!" Tom was stalking me during the divorce process. One day, he even called me at my attorney's office, and my attorney handed me the phone! Tom was across the highway and needed a ride somewhere. I gave him a ride. I shouldn't have, but I did.

Tom was fighting me for joint custody, and I wasn't about to give it to him, especially when at one of our ecumenical counseling sessions, he had been diagnosed by the test results as bipolar. I ended up giving him custody—after he took my daughter across the states one Christmas. She was middle school-aged. Tom manipulated her into calling me and saying over the phone that she wasn't going to tell me where they were and that she was not coming back until I agreed to joint custody. A few months later, my attorney said, "Let's just give him joint custody."

Venting to friends and family became therapeutic for me. Before that, I felt that I needed to be loyal to my husband and I shouldn't be talking about him in a negative light. I'm especially grateful for my brother-in-law and sister-in-law who were both good Christians; they were there for me. My siblings became a source of comfort and support. There's a special couple that I've known since high school. I know they were praying for me. Years later one of them said to me, "You were married to the devil, weren't you, Carol?" Even a stranger was uplifting—a lock man—when he said to me, "Don't you dare give that man the new set of keys." Tom had berated me while this lock man was changing my locks. Which, ultimately, Tom manipulated the kids anyway—they gave him a set of keys!

Our marriage lasted for fifteen years—until the bitter end. A couple of years into our divorce, Tom lost another business and lost the two houses. Tom decided to move out of state, took our daughter, and left our son behind; he said he didn't want him. Prior to leaving, Tom created a big scene. I went into the kitchen with our daughter and asked her if there was something going on that shouldn't be happening between her and her dad. She said no. I had been concerned and had mentioned it to my attorney that she was twelve, and Tom was allowing her to sleep in the same bed with him. Of course, my attorney didn't address the issue, even though I was paying his attorney fees.

Our son eventually went to live with Tom anyway. During the kids' middle school years, I felt like Tom had kidnapped them; I had no idea where they lived. I contacted my attorney who did plumb nothing for me. Tom wouldn't allow the kids to call me or visit. If they did, it would be very sporadic, but they wouldn't let me know where they were. At one point, Tom decided to let them come live with me. The kids would take turns and go back and forth.

Tom always told the kids that if they didn't come back to him, he would kill himself. During our son's high school graduation, Tom showed up. Tom acted arrogant, had a narcissistic attitude, and then left. Our daughter asked Tom, her dad, to give her away when she got married, but he refused to because he was not allowed to stay in the same hotel that our friends and family were staying. Tom did not want to stay at a separate hotel. My children have said as adults (individually) that they wish they had stayed and lived with me the whole time.

I waited at least a year and a half after the divorce before I dated anyone. I kept saying to myself and others that it was too soon. I needed to heal. I used the alone times to draw closer to Jesus Who had been calling me since middle school, but I was always too busy, never had a desire, or I was too messed up in my marriage. I recommitted my life to Jesus during that time and began to read the Bible, prayed, and went back to attending church. I would journal my prayers in spiral notebooks; it was very therapeutic. I knew the Holy Spirit was ministering to me. I got better—*He* got me through it. Once in a while, I would go out because I like to country western dance. A few girlfriends and I would go out and line dance. I liked doing that.

One day, my sister-in-law invited me to her church and suggested that I meet this guy, Matt, who taught the singles Sunday school class. I noticed a lot of women were hanging on him, so I thought, "I don't need that!" I church-hopped for a year after that (looking for a man). Then I returned to my sister-in-law's church. I decided to commit to this church and to attend for the right reason—Jesus. Matt called me one night to go country western dancing with him. I was glad, but I was hesitant (even though I had been praying for a *real* Christian man to come into my life). Once a Christian man came into my life, I didn't know what to do with him! Matt came from a stable Lutheran family; he was raised with a close extended family. Matt's parents were married for almost fifty years until his mother passed.

After a few months of dating, Matt declared, "I think I'm falling in love with you." By Christmas, we were telling everyone that we were going to get married. We got married that summer. I had been divorced about three years, and so had Matt. Matt's former wife had divorced him (after her multiple affairs throughout their marriage). Most of the church body knew about his sixteen years of marriage and her infidelity. I felt that I could trust his reason for their divorce. Once I remarried, Tom pretty much stopped reappearing to abuse me.

Matt and I have been married for twenty-four years. My relationship with Matt is different because we have Jesus in our marriage. Matt's a wonderful man; he is gentle, loving, and kind. During our sixth year of marriage, I was diagnosed with breast cancer. Matt was marvelous when I met him for lunch and I gave him the news. One evening before praying over our meal, he told me that if he could take my cancer treatments for me, he would. This meant a whole lot to me. Matt saw me through it, and I wasn't the best patient. At times, I could be very angry or anxious. I could be all kinds of ways (even be angry at *him*), and he took it calmly, supported me all the way through, and I love him for it! I took medicine for fourteen years after the surgery, and I'm still cancer-free, *praise the Lord*.

After leaving my abusive relationship, my life has become a life of peace and calmness; I no longer wait for something to explode. I don't have to deal with the constant anger and the hateful stuff that used to spew out all the time. Matt has never treated me that way—but my adult children occasionally do. Granted, my daughter is stronger and better able to deal with life because of all that she has been through (she's not naïve like I was), and that's a plus.

However, there are still days where both my daughter and son will let their anger get the best of them. My adult children don't know Jesus, so they're still not there in dealing with their anger. Once in a while, they attempt to stomp on my spiritual beliefs, but I won't let them. My daughter has a steady job as a nurse. My son has had the most difficulties making it in life and has been homeless; he has a seven-year-old son that is being raised by his wife. It's as if he has vanished off the globe; he's unable to hold down a job and moves from place to place, manipulating and controlling others to get what he needs or wants.

My past life was oppressive and horrible. There were some good times, but when it was bad, it was very, very bad! My life was totally out of control. Now it's an exciting life, full of blessings. I wish that I would have responded to Jesus' calling sooner than I did because it just makes such a difference in my life. I understand now how He wants me to live and that my past life did not honor Him. I wish I wouldn't have been so tied to the world and the things of the world. I was fortunate that I had a support system in place when I went through my abusive relationship. I would say to anyone who finds that they're in an abusive relationship (even if their support has been destroyed), get a support system—and *get out*!

ENDNOTES

PART I SPIRIT MIND BODY
1. Daniel J. Siegel, M.D., Begley (2007); Doidge (2007); Kempermann et al. (2002). *The Developing Mind: How Relationships and the Brain Interact to Shape Who We Are*, 2nd ed. (New York: The Guilford Press, 2012) 253-254, 419.
2. Ibid.
3. Daniel J. Siegel, M.D., Hall and Lifshitz (2010); Thompson et al. (2009); Doidge (2007). *The Developing Mind: How Relationships and the Brain Interact to Shape Who We Are*, 2nd ed. (New York: The Guilford Press, 2012) 254, 419.
4. Andrew Newberg, M.D. and Mark Robert Waldman, *How God Changes Your Brain: Breakthrough Findings from a Leading Neuroscientist* (New York: Ballantine Books, 2010) 4, 7, 41, 63.

RESOURCES

The National Domestic Violence Hotline
1-800-799-7233 1-800-799-SAFE Toll-Free
www.ndvh.org
www.thehotline.org

Domestic Shelters
Free national database of domestic violence shelter programs.
www.domesticshelters.org

Break the Cycle
202-824-0707
www.breakthecycle.org

Break the Silence (BTSADV)
1-800-855-BTS (1777)
Mon-Sun. Supportive assistance and connection to resources.
www.breakthesilencedv.org

Final Salute, Inc.
Mission: To provide homeless women Veterans with safe and suitable housing.
One of the factors contributing to female veteran homelessness is domestic violence.
703-224-8845
https://www.finalsaluteinc.org

Military OneSource
800-342-9647 (U.S. or Overseas)
TTY/TDD: Dial 711 and give the toll-free number 800-342-9647
https://www.militaryonesource.mil/
 24/7/365 abuse helpline via telephone or on website, click on Confidential Help in the menu; live chat with a prompt response is available for all electronic devices.
To locate resources at your military installation go to: https://installations.militaryonesource.mil/

Women's Law
www.womenslaw.org
Provides civilian and military domestic violence information and laws.

National Military Family Association
2800 Eisenhower Avenue, Suite 250
Alexandria, VA 22314
703-931-6632
info@MilitaryFamily.org

Operation We are Here
Resource Center for the Military & its Supporters
Email: opwearehere@gmail.com
www.operationwearehere.com

The Mary Kay Foundation for Domestic Abuse
Mary Kay sponsored text-for-help line (for victim or if you know a victim that needs help).
Text "loveis" to 22522

HOPE for the Heart Care Center
Prayer & Christian Counseling referral source.
Hope care representatives are available M-F 24 hrs.
1-800-488-4673 1-800-488- HOPE 4673 Toll-Free

RESOURCES

Americans Overseas Domestic Violence Crisis Center
International Toll-Free (24/7)
1-866-USWOMEN 1-866-879-6636 Toll-Free
www.866uswomen.org

National Teen Dating Abuse Helpline
1-866-331-9474 Toll-Free
www.loveisrespect.org

Childhelp USA/National Child Abuse Hotline
1-800-422-4453 1-800-4-A-CHILD Toll-Free
www.childhelpusa.org www.childhelp.org

World Childhood Foundation Inc.
Mission: To stimulate, promote and enable the development of solutions to prevent and address sexual abuse, exploitation, and violence against children.
900 3rd Ave. 29th Floor
New York, NY 10022
212-867-6088
Website:info@childhood-USA.org

Rape, Abuse, & Incest National Network
1-800- 656-4673 1-800-656- HOPE Toll-Free
www.rainn.org

National Human Trafficking Resource Center/Polaris Project
Call: 1-888-373-7888 Toll-Free Text: HELP to Be Free (233733)
www.polarisproject.org

Battered Women's Justice Project
1-800-903-0111
www.bwjp.org

Brain Injury Resource Center
P.O.BOX 84151
Seattle, WA 98124-5451
206-621-8558
Email: %20brain@headinjury.com
www.headinjury.com

Deaf Abused Women's Network (DAWN)
One in two deaf women experience family violence.
One in three deaf women is a victim of sexual assault.
Email: Hotline@deafdawn.org
VP: 202-559-5366
www.deafdawn.org

Abused Deaf Women's Advocacy Services (ADWAS)
Email: Deafhelp@thehotline.org
VP: 1-855-812-1000 Toll-Free

American Bar Association Commission on Domestic Violence
1-202-662-1000
www.abanet.org/domviol

ASPIRE News
An app that is hidden in a traditional news reader icon with cryptic programming capability.
Smartphone App Offers Resource Contacts & Help for Victims of Abuse: The victim can program the app to alert "trusted personal contacts/resources" of the victim's emergency status.
https://www.whengeorgiasmiled.org/the-aspire-news-app/

RESOURCES

NNEDV
National Network to End Domestic Violence
1325 Massachusetts Ave NW 7th Floor
Washington, DC 20005-4188
202-543-5566
www.techsafety.org

In order to maintain victim safety and privacy through the proper software, The National Network to End Domestic Violence (NNEDV) Safety Net Project, together with the Office for Victims of Crime, Office of Justice Programs, U.S. Department of Justice provide guidance on a Digital Services Toolkit to protect victims from digital abuse. The toolkit is equipped with resources for local programs that offer services via text, chat, video call, and other digital technologies.

TracFone Wireless, Inc.
A pre-paid mobile phone network operating in the U.S., Puerto Rico, and the U.S. Virgin Islands, who also offers several other cellphone brands with services from various phone companies. Monday-Sunday 8:00 a.m.-11:45 p.m. Eastern Standard Time 1-800-867-7183 0r 1-880-378-9575 Press # 4 then repeatedly ask for customer service when the prompts do not apply to you. If the prompts ask for your TracFone # or other information which you do not have, say "other" and a representative will answer.
www.tracfone.com

OTHER BOOKS BY REINA DAVISON

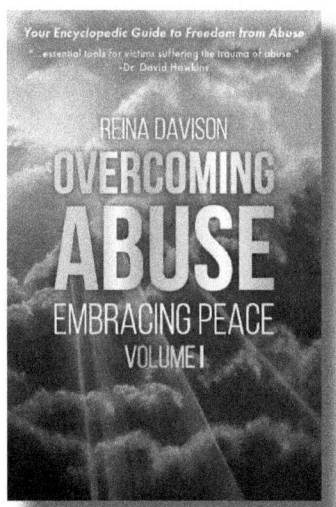

Overcoming Abuse: Embracing Peace Volume I Your Encyclopedic Guide to Freedom from Abuse arms victims and their support system with a body of knowledge on the trauma of abuse. Victim abuse has historically and up to the present been treated as a mere societal botheration and remains predominantly an unapproachable enigma. Problem-solving clinical faith-based strategies are provided for victims and our society in order that they may experience abuse-free lives. Self-told testimonial stories of triumphant victims that have overcome their abuse are revealed; as the victim is guided to overcome her own abuse. The result: As an overcomer of her abuse—she embraces peace and becomes—the woman God intended her to be! To bring the message of *Overcoming Abuse: Embracing Peace Volume I* to your organization, church, or event, visit: www.overcomingabuse.info

Overcoming Abuse: Embracing Peace Volume III An Encyclopedic Guide for Helpers of Abuse Victims is a guidebook that brings to light the historical gravity of the problem—victim abuse. De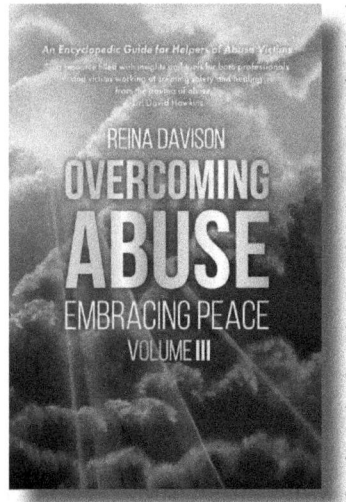tailed treatment strategies are provided through clinical and faith-based approaches for the victim and those interested in helping the victim in civilian and/or military jurisdiction. Case scenario self-told stories of triumphant victims that have overcome their abuse are cited. Interventions for the victim of trauma are circumscribed: including working with the immediate needs of the victim, assisting with safety decisions, modeling trust and self-protection, dealing with victim regression, using cognitive behavioral and reality therapy, neurological interventions, and treating PTSD. To bring the message of ***Overcoming Abuse: Embracing Peace Volume III*** to your organization, church, or event, visit: **www.overcomingabuse.info**

OTHER BOOKS BY REINA DAVISON

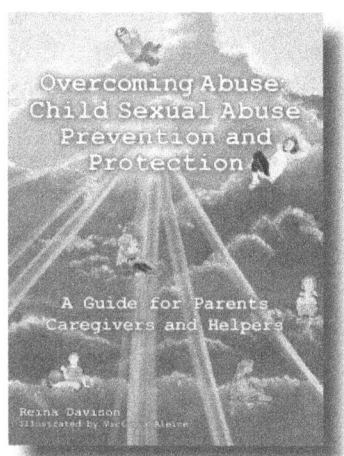

Overcoming Abuse: Child Sexual Abuse Prevention and Protection: A Guide for Parents Caregivers and Helpers is a parent's handbook to learn the dynamics of Child Sexual Abuse (CSA), the sex offender profile, and *how* to prevent and protect a child from being a target of CSA anywhere, including the internet. This book guides the adult on initiating conversation to help the child gain an understanding about the precious gift of his body; and walks the adult through introducing a healthy, age-appropriate, biblical perspective on human sexuality. The concept of overcoming Child Sexual Abuse is fully addressed to encourage and strengthen the parent/caregiver and child as they come together to empower the child against CSA (whether he/she has never experienced CSA or has already been a target).

To bring the message of *Overcoming Abuse: Child Sexual Abuse Prevention and Protection* to your organization, church, or event, visit: **www.overcomingabuse.info**

Overcoming Abuse: My Body Belongs to God and Me A Child's Body Safety Guide is a book written for a parent, caregiver, or helper to read to children from pre-school to fifth grade. Trusted adults can teach children how to identify *no touch people* and how to distinguish "good touch" (God touch) from "no touch" in a non-frightening way and non-threatening environment. A series of possible scenarios with no touch people (including the internet) are presented, and the child is guided as to how to respond in a similar situation. The child is emboldened to stay away from no touch people and is strengthened and encouraged that most touch *is* good touch!

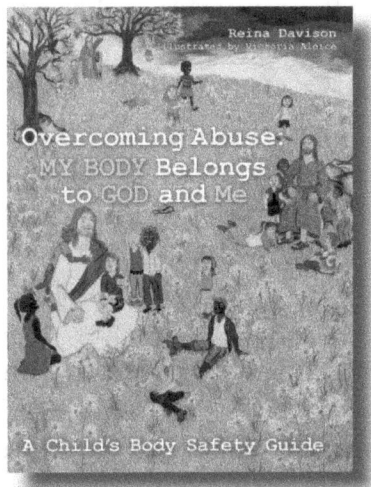

To bring the message of ***Overcoming Abuse: My Body Belongs to God and Me*** to your organization, church, or event, visit: **www.overcomingabuse.info**

www.ingramcontent.com/pod-product-compliance
Lightning Source LLC
Chambersburg PA
CBHW050104170426
43198CB00014B/2453